Evidence-Based Pressure Ulcer Prevention

A STUDY GUIDE FOR NURSES

Karen S. Clay, RN, BSN, CWCN

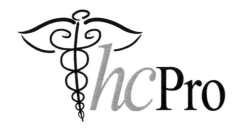

Evidence-Based Pressure Ulcer Prevention: A Study Guide for Nurses is published by HCPro, Inc.

HCPro, Inc., provides information resources for the healthcare industry.

Karen S. Clay, RN, BSN, CWCN, Author

Jackie Diehl Singer, Graphic Artist

Barbara Acello, RN, MSN, Contributor

Crystal Beland, Layout Artist

Lisa Frizzell, RN, CWCN, COCN, Contributor/Reviewer

Jean St. Pierre, Creative Director

Melanie Roberts, Associate Editor

D. René Molina, Cover Designer

Emily Sheahan, Executive Editor

Kathryn Levesque, Group Publisher

Lauren Rubenzahl, Copy Editor

Suzanne Perney, Publisher

Steve DeGrappo, Cover Design

Advice given is general. Readers should consult professional counsel for specific legal, ethical, or clinical questions.

Arrangements can be made for quantity discounts. For more information, contact:

HCPro, Inc.

200 Hoods Lane

P.O. Box 1168

Marblehead, MA 01945

Telephone: 800/650-6787 or 781/639-1872

Fax: 781/639-2982

E-mail: *customerservice@hcpro.com*

Visit HCPro, Inc., at its World Wide Web sites:

www.hcpro.com and *www.hcmarketplace.com*

CONTENTS

Contents

- Define "pressure ulcer" and explain the role of impaired blood supply in the creation of pressure ulcers

- Identify two influences that put patients at risk for pressure ulcers and that may be beyond the care-givers' control

- Define the "rule of 30," and explain where on the body pressure is prevented by using this rule

- Identify two reasons why heels are the second most common sites of pressure ulcers and provide an example of how to "off-load" pressure from this area

- List and explain the four pressure ulcer stages

- Define "backstaging" and explain why it is *not* recommended

- Identify the two most widely used risk-assessment tools, and list two of the subscales covered by each tool

- List four intrinsic and extrinsic risk factors for pressure ulcer development

- List and identify the four types of tissue to be observed in a pressure ulcer

- Identify the three-dimensional measurement formula, and list two related measurement techniques

- State three possible strategies nurses can perform to relieve pain during dressing changes

- Identify and differentiate the three possible microbiologic states within pressure ulcers

- Define "MVTR," and identify good and bad MVTR

- List the seven "rights" to consider when performing dressing changes

- List two wound-care products that promote a moist wound environment

- Define "negative pressure wound therapy," and list two factors to consider about the patient before administering this therapy

- Identify and explain the three parameters the PUSH tool is designed to monitor

- List the three factors that must be consistently addressed prior to identifying a wound as "recalcitrant"

- Explain why taking creative liberties with physician-ordered treatments is a bad practice, and give one specific example of this occurence from your work setting in nursing

- Identify two care-plan risk factors, and explain how they affect risk or healing

- Explain why proper, detailed documentation is important when defending pressure ulcer-related lawsuits

- List three aspects of risk and care about which primary caregivers, patients, families, and other professional staff should be educated

Background and Scope

The Wound, Ostomy and Continence Nurses (WOCN) Society estimates that more than 1 million people develop pressure ulcers every year and that an estimated 1.5–3 million U.S. adults currently receive treatment for pressure ulcers.[1]

However, the actual scope of the pressure ulcer problem is unknown because not all healthcare settings are required to report such statistics.

In this context, the prevalence of pressure ulcers indicates the percentage of patients with them—such as those in a hospital, nursing home, or certain hospital unit—at one point in time in a specific population. In 2001, the National Pressure Ulcer Advisory Panel (NPUAP) estimated that the prevalence of pressure ulcers in acute care ranged from 10.1% to 17%; in long-term care, the prevalence ranged from 2.3% to 28%.[2]

These data conclude that pressure ulcers are generally less prevalent in acute-care settings.

Incidence rates, however, tell a different story. Such rates indicate the percentage of patients who developed pressure ulcers *after* admission to that setting. Incidence rates better reflect the effectiveness of a healthcare facility's pressure ulcer prevention program than do numbers reflecting the prevalence of pressure ulcers. NPUAP data from 2001 indicate that incidence rates in acute-care facilities ranged from 0.4% to 38% at that time; in long-term care, they ranged from 2.2% to 23.9%.[2]

These data make sense. Acute-care facilities tend to have fewer pressure ulcer cases due to both shorter stays and the physiology of pressure ulcers, including how they reveal themselves. The WOCN guideline reports that pressure ulcers may take as long as five days to present themselves.[1] Thus, a patient may not remain in the acute-care setting long enough for a pressure ulcer to become visible.

But this is not always the case. Acute-care facilities may receive from long-term care or other settings patients who have pressure ulcers that must be treated. Such care involves expenses that are necessary but difficult to quantify.

The financial cost of pressure ulcers is difficult to determine because reported treatment costs account for many different variables and, therefore, are not comparable. For example, some studies include all costs (i.e., nursing care, physician fees, supplies, and room) while others include only direct costs (e.g., supplies, medications). Despite this lack of consistency in measurement, it is generally agreed that expenses for patients with pressure ulcers are exceptionally higher than expenses for those without. Pressure ulcers cost $2.2–$3.6 billion in the U.S. acute-care setting.[3] And, in addition to the direct costs of pressure ulcers, patients with them are more likely to develop healthcare-associated infections and other complications, further driving up their cost of care.

What is a pressure ulcer?

In 2003, the WOCN defined a pressure ulcer as "any lesion caused by unrelieved pressure resulting in damage of underlying tissue. Pressure ulcers are usually located over bony prominences and are staged to classify the degree of damage observed."

It is important to understand the role of impaired blood supply in the creation of pressure ulcers. Although the initial insult is indeed pressure, the underlying pathophysiologic changes are related to the impairment of capillary blood flow. Such impairment can cause a cascade of events, including cellular and muscle responses.

Cellular response

At each stage of this cascade, other pathophysiologic changes can occur at the cellular level, including damage to the epithelium, platelet activation, tissue acidosis, and alteration in lymphatic flow. See Figure 1.1 for a chart of cellular responses.

Muscle response

Although the visible damage to the skin's surface is a concern, the real problem is the muscle damage,

---

FIGURE 1.1 | **Chart of Cellular Responses**

Pressure → capillary occlusion/blood vessel damage → tissue hypoxia

If pressure is relieved
↓
↓
Reactive hyperemia (blanching erythema)
↓
Hypoxia resolves

If pressure continues
↓
↓
Tissue ischemia
↓
↓
↓
Nutrients and metabolic wastes accumulate
↓
Capillary damage and leakage of fluid in interstitial space (= edema)
↓
Tissue edema causes slower perfusion
↓
PRESSURE ULCER

---

which is not initially evident. Researchers have long understood that pressure is highest at the point of contact between the bony prominence and the muscle fascia. The deep-tissue damage that such pressure can cause is far more significant than skin impairment, and there is often little external evidence (at the skin-surface level) of the injury that lies beneath. In pressure ulcer development, visible skin damage is the tip of the iceberg.

Indeed, deep-pressure ulcers begin to form at the bone and *then* extend to the skin—and the pressure at the bone is three to five times higher than at the skin.[4] See Figure 1.2 for an example of an inverted cone/pressure gradient that depicts the more extensive damage at the muscle/bone.

Nurses must understand this pressure gradient when assessing a wound. When damage is present at the skin level, carefully inspect the area for evidence of deeper tissue damage.

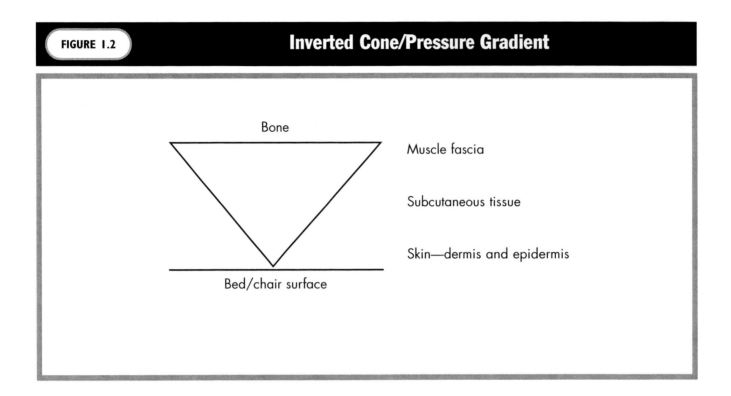

FIGURE 1.2 — Inverted Cone/Pressure Gradient

Bone

Muscle fascia

Subcutaneous tissue

Skin—dermis and epidermis

Bed/chair surface

Tissue tolerance and the 'blame game'

The intensity and duration of pressure are important factors in pressure ulcer development. High-intensity pressure—in this case, the weight of the patient—can cause tissue damage over a short period of time, but low-intensity pressure caused by prolonged immobility, decreased sensory perception inadequate nutrition over a long period of time can cause tissue injury as well. Tissue tolerance—that is, how much pressure the skin can tolerate—is another important factor in pressure ulcer development.

In her book, *Acute & Chronic Wounds*, Ruth A. Bryant, RN, MS, CWOCN, reports on an experiment that showed that deep-tissue ischemia can occur without any manifestation at the skin level and that subsequent small amounts of pressure may result in breakdown of the skin.[5] The researcher applied pressure of 100 mm Hg to rat muscle for two hours and found no evidence of trauma. Three days later, he applied half the pressure (50 mm Hg) to the same tissue for half the time (one hour). The rat muscle then showed evidence of damage. The experiment demonstrated that muscle damage occurred during the second application of pressure, even though the intensity and duration of the pressure were half those of the initial application.

The moral of the story is two-fold: Damage is not always evident with the initial insult, and it actually may occur in the midst of properly applied therapeutic interventions at short duration and with pressure reduction. The implication for nursing staff: Stop the "blame game." It is not uncommon to hear nurses on Monday mornings exclaim, "They must not have repositioned her this weekend because her skin was fine on Friday and now she has a pressure ulcer." The reality may be that on Thursday the intensity and duration of pressure were high and that a change occurred on the weekend despite application of care-planned interventions.

The price of pressure ulcer prevention

Interestingly, pressure ulcer prevention programs are estimated to cost $60,000 at onset, with subsequent annual costs of $10,000.[6] These figures include the cost of training and of creating policies and procedures, and they vary based on equipment purchases. One implication is clear: It costs less both fiscally and in human suffering to prevent pressure ulcers than it does to treat them.

State, federal, and JCAHO requirements

According to the Social Security Act §1861, at-risk patients should be identified in the admission assessment, and discharge planning should be started the day of hospital admission. Doing so not only is mandated by law but also provides for continuity of care.

"The hospital must identify, at an early stage of hospitalization, those patients who are likely to suffer adverse health consequences upon discharge in the absence of adequate discharge planning."[7] Staff should work closely with the patient and the patient's caregivers to ensure that the protocols (e.g., specific dressing instructions, nutrition, pressure-reducing surface) initiated as an inpatient are continued post-discharge.

Payment is another issue affected by your hospital's pressure ulcer prevention efforts. For instance, the Medicare payment system for hospitals was set by Section 1886(d) of the Social Security Act. Payments to hospitals for Medicare-eligible patients fall under Medicare Part A (hospital insurance), and individual cases are placed in categories such as Diagnostic-Related Groups (DRG). Each DRG has a payment assigned to it based on the average cost to treat a patient in that group. Therefore, with fixed DRG payment, it makes sense to diligently focus efforts on assessment and prevention of pressure ulcers before they ever begin.

Lawsuits are another reason to practice pressure ulcer prevention actively. If you deviate from state and federal requirements and thus place the patient at risk of pressure ulcer development, you also put the organization (and individual practitioners) at risk of being sued for negligence. Negligence is failure to act as a reasonable, prudent person in the protection and care of another. It is also failure to meet the standards of care, which are the norm for practice and may stem from usual and customary practice, federal and state law, professional associations, and policies of the organization.

Healthcare providers can prevail under this scrutiny when clinical records show that they consistently adhered to the standard of care for pressure ulcers and when records reflect that disease processes or complications made pressure ulcer development more likely. In addition, the hospital must show that it has a comprehensive staff education program on the prevention and treatment of pressure ulcers.

For accredited hospitals, such as those certified by the Joint Commission on Accreditation of Healthcare Organizations (JCAHO)—which measures healthcare organizations against national standards set by health professionals—there is flexibility in pressure ulcer care practices as long as standards of care and regulations are being met.

Organizational policy and procedures

Along with following the state, federal, and JCAHO requirements regarding pressure ulcer prevention and management, you must also adhere to the policies and procedures of your hospital. These policies and procedures are the foundation of pressure ulcer prevention and management programs and serve as a blueprint for the interdisciplinary team. If your organization's policies are solid and based on accepted standards, they provide a good framework for nursing practice and interdisciplinary involvement; they also provide the opportunity to establish team goals and to document the organizational commitment and philosophy. Therefore, it is vital to adhere to your hospital's policies and procedures if your main goal is to administer effective, appropriate care to your patients who have or are at risk for developing pressure ulcers.

Views on pressure ulcer prevention

Some experts believe all pressure ulcers are preventable, but not all share this belief; some experts believe there can be influences beyond the caregivers' control. These influences can range from patient noncompliance to end-of-life directives that require a different goal of care. For example, if a patient refuses to participate in range-of-motion exercises, physical therapy assistance with ambulation, or repositioning activities, you may not be able to prevent pressure ulcers from forming. Some patients refuse repositioning and will not allow pressure-relief mattresses or wheelchair cushions despite caregiver education. Thus, your hands may be tied despite your best efforts.

In the case of terminal care, your patient may not accept any food or may have advance directives that prohibit artificial feeding. Perhaps pain limits repositioning—and with comfort as the primary goal, a frequent repositioning schedule may be inappropriate. Both the absence of proper nutrition and less frequent repositioning increase a patient's likelihood of developing a pressure ulcer. Although these influences are the exception rather than the rule, they nonetheless are part of the equation.

Pressure ulcer prevention is a complex task that requires the critical thinking and coordinated activities of an interdisciplinary team. In many cases, pressure ulcer development is related to the quality of care provided—and we need to embrace this reality.

References

1. Wound, Ostomy and Continence Nurse Society. 2003. Guideline for prevention and management of pressure ulcers. Glenview, IL: WOCN.

2. National Pressure Ulcer Advisory Panel. Cuddigan J., E.A. Ayeloo, and C. Sussman, eds. 2001. Pressure ulcers in America: Prevalence, incidence, and implications for the future. Reston, VA: NPUAP.

3. Beckrich, K., and S. Aronovitch. 1999. Hospital-acquired pressure ulcers: A comparison of costs in medical vs. surgical patients. *Nursing Economics* 17(5): 263–271.

4. Shea, J.D. 1975. Pressure sores: classification and management. *Clinical Orthopedics* 112(10): 89–100.

5. Bryant, R. 2000. *Acute and chronic wounds.* St. Louis, MO: Mosby, Inc. 231–232.

6. Moore, S.M., and L. Wise. 1997. Reducing nonsocomial pressure ulcers. *Journal of Nursing Administration* 27(10): 28.

7. Compilation of the Social Security Laws. *www.ssa.gov/OP_Home/ssact/title18/1861.htm* (Accessed on March 26, 2005.)

To create an effective program for pressure ulcer prevention, first conduct a risk assessment to identify risk factors, and then focus your prevention program on minimizing their negative effects. When addressing pressure ulcers as a risk-management problem, prevention is the number one solution. It alleviates needless patient suffering, unnecessary healthcare costs, and associated litigation. This focus will include management of pressure, friction, shear, moisture, and any other individual risk factors.

Positioning

Frequent positioning of the patient can help prevent capillary occlusion, which leads to tissue ischemia and pressure ulcers. Pressure ulcers form due to the combination of the intensity of pressure and the duration of pressure, and although repositioning will not reduce the intensity of pressure, it will reduce duration, which is more critical.

The Agency for Healthcare Research and Quality (AHRQ), formerly the Agency for Health Care Policy and Research, recommends repositioning at least every two hours.[1] However, the frequency of repositioning required to prevent ischemia depends on capillary-closing pressures, which vary by person and pressure point. For an example, say you work on a 40-bed unit with 30 at-risk patients who require repositioning a minimum of every two hours (i.e., 12 times per day). This equates to 360 turns a day, or 120 turns every shift, or 15 turns per hour. As you can see, this task is enormous.

It is difficult to meet repositioning requirements even under normal circumstances and with full staffing, so envision trying to reposition patients properly while short-staffed or during a shift that schedules fewer staff. In addition, repositioning often accompanies incontinence care, which requires more staff time and occurs in the midst of assisting with morning or evening care, showers, rehabilitation/activity schedules, and meals. Therefore, it is difficult for staff to provide proper care without adequate staffing.

No matter what the staffing circumstances, use the "rule of 30" when repositioning patients. This rule indicates that you should elevate the head of the bed to 30° or less and that the body, when repositioned to either side, should be placed in a 30° laterally inclined position. In this position, the patient's hips and shoulders are tilted 30° from supine, which prevents pressure over the trochanter and sacrum. If the head of the bed is elevated beyond 30°, limit the duration of this position to minimize shear forces and pressure.

Use positioning pillows, pads, or foam wedges to keep bony prominences from direct contact with one another. Also use them for patients with splints or multipodus boots, which could create significant pressure should they come in contact with an unprotected opposing limb. Doing so will help to maintain proper body alignment and reduce the potential of pressure ulcer formation from bone-to-bone contact. See Figure 2.1 for an illustration of the proper use of positioning pillows.

FIGURE 2.1   **Proper Use of Positioning Pillows**

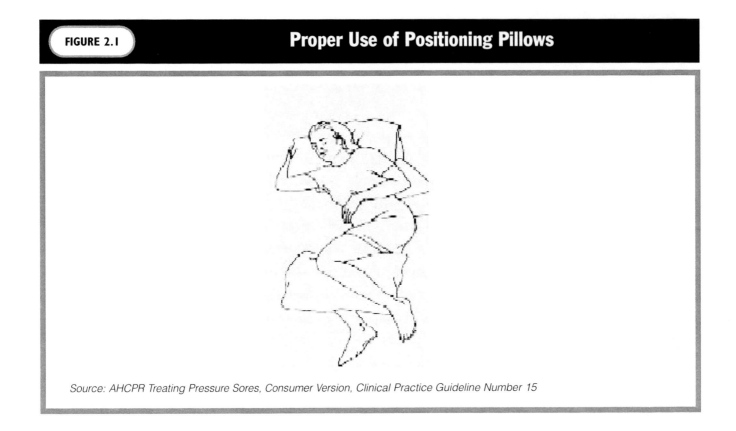

Source: AHCPR Treating Pressure Sores, Consumer Version, Clinical Practice Guideline Number 15

Contractures

Contracture prevention and management of contractures are important not only for their own sake but also for preventing pressure ulcers. Contractures, which cause shortened and flexed positions of the affected area, develop in predictable patterns, so splinting, range-of-motion exercises, and proper positioning can help prevent their occurrence. Such prevention is necessary not only because of the loss of strength and function contractures cause, but also because they may compromise positioning and hygiene. In addition, significantly contracted limbs are thought to result in impaired blood supply to that limb—which should raise a red flag, as pressure ulcer development has its origins in impaired blood flow and resultant tissue ischemia. Although a contracture will not necessarily result in a pressure ulcer, healing of any pressure ulcer that does erupt will be complicated by the poor perfusion of the limb.

Repositioning clocks

Some hospitals use repositioning clocks to monitor repositioning schedules. The basic concept is that a clock placed at the bedside prescribes a particular position at a specific time (e.g., 10:00 left side, 12:00 back, or 2:00 right side, etc.). Theoretically, it is easier for supervisors to detect whether a patient's repositioning schedule is being adhered to if they see that at 10:00 all at-risk patients will be positioned on their left sides.

Although the intent of the clock—which is to guide every two-hour repositioning—is good, some experts do not regularly recommend its use. Instead, they suggest designing positioning schedules with an individual patient's needs and preferences in mind, which is important in maintaining patient compliance with interventions. In addition, prescriptive clocks do not address the needs of a patient with limited turning surfaces. If a patient has a sacral pressure ulcer, for example, you may not want to include the supine (back) position in your repositioning regimen because you want to keep the sacral area totally off-loaded. Use positioning clocks judiciously and always in the context of your patients' individualized needs and preferences.

Although patients may be capable of independent position changes, they may not remember to make them. For example, an alert and oriented patient with paraplegia might use trapeze equipment for bed mobility and might independently transfer to a wheelchair. Although capable of this mobility, however, the sensation (i.e., discomfort) associated with the need to reposition is absent. An alarm watch can be helpful for such a patient. Set the watch for two-hour intervals to cue this capable patient to reposition himself or herself.

Repositioning does not always entail a full turn from left side to right side or from back to left side. It may be helpful to intervene with small, frequent position changes using pillows, bath blankets, and wedges to reduce pressure. These changes expand the weight-bearing surface by molding to the body and minimizing point pressure.

For positioning of chair-bound patients, pay attention to their anatomy, postural alignment, distribution of weight, and support of the feet.[1] A small shift may be as easy as elevating the legs. In addition, standing and reseating the patient in the chair interrupts the increase in pressure from the duration and gravity of pressure that occurs over time. If patients can reposition themselves, encourage them to do chair push-ups at 15-minute intervals.

Staff often lose or neglect the use of wheelchair legs and footrests. Although it is common for rehabilitation staff to search for the leg rests assigned to a particular patient and wheelchair, nursing staff do not always share this concern. But they should. This equipment not only maintains postural alignment but also may play a significant role in pressure reduction. Nurses must be sensitized to this problem and understand that although the hospital may have provided the best possible pressure-reducing wheelchair cushion, the effects of the cushion are minimal in the absence of foot rests, with the patients' legs dangling.

Heels

Heels pose a significant risk for pressure ulcer development. They are the second most common sites of pressure ulcers (after the sacrum) in the supine position. Because heels have small surface areas and underlying bony surfaces, redistribution of pressure is nearly impossible. Heels also have lower resting blood-perfusion levels, which are compounded by the fact that many elderly patients have compromised lower-extremity blood flow.

Beyond regularly scheduled pressure risk assessments, assess a patient's potential for heel-ulcer formation when he or she has an acute change in status. Heel ulcers often develop when there is just a brief change in mobility, such as when a patient falls and sustains a hip bruise. The patient may be less mobile for a few days either because of a sore hip or because he or she is on bed-rest awaiting the results of an x-ray. In both cases, heel pressure ulcers may develop quickly, so it is important to initiate preventive activities.

Most support surfaces cannot adequately reduce the interface pressure under the heels. Thus, there are a few types of "zero pressure" three-cell alternating-therapy support surfaces that will eliminate heel pressure in 7 1/2-minute cycles. There are also commercially available heel-lift products that range from high-density foam blocks/boots to multipodus boots. When using these products, nurses must assess the fit and provide close, ongoing monitoring to ensure that irritation and pressure do not occur at another site on the lower extremity. The most effective intervention, however, is total "off-loading" of the heel by elevating the lower extremities on a pillow (see Figure 2.2).

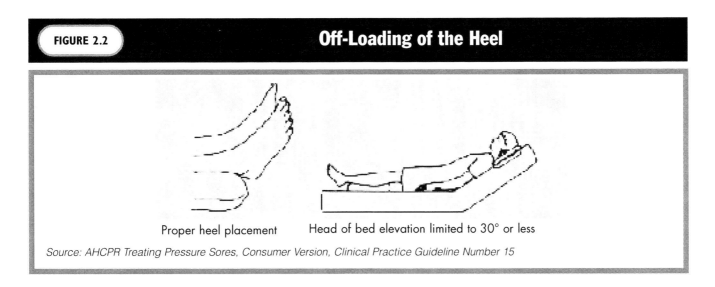

FIGURE 2.2	**Off-Loading of the Heel**

Proper heel placement · Head of bed elevation limited to 30° or less

Source: AHCPR Treating Pressure Sores, Consumer Version, Clinical Practice Guideline Number 15

Contrary to popular belief, "bunny boots" do not provide pressure relief. These boots, made of soft or quilted cotton, may afford some protection from friction, but they do not relieve pressure. In patients with very sensitive skin or at extremely high risk of pressure ulcer development, problems may develop at the seams even of new and well-maintained cloth bunny boots. If bunny boots are going to be used to minimize friction, consider using those made of high-density seamless foam.

Bed linens

Assess bed linens for their impact on pressure ulcer development. Years ago, in nursing school, students were required to make "foot pleats" at the bottom of the bed when making it. They ensured that the linens were not too tight at the base of the bed. Both in practice and in theory, it made sense to do so in order to reduce pressure on the heels: If you envision a patient lying supine in a freshly made bed, you will realize that the patient's feet and heels maybe compressed to the bed by tight linens. Thus, even if you don't make foot pleats, relieve pressure on the feet by loosening the sheets at the foot of the bed when assisting a patient back to bed or by using a foot cradle.

Support surfaces

A cornerstone in reducing pressure is choosing support surfaces, such as pressure-reducing cushions, mattresses (e.g., high-density foam, gel, etc.), and specialty beds or mattress-replacement systems. The intent of these products is to reduce "interface pressure," forces that act between the body and the support surface and are primarily affected by the composition of the body tissue, the stiffness of the support surface, and characteristics of the patient's body.

Interface pressure is different than capillary-closing pressure, although there is often confusion between these two concepts. Capillary-closing pressure describes the minimal amount of pressure required to collapse a capillary, which causes tissue anoxia. Commonly, capillary pressures are considered to be 32 mm Hg, but in reality, they vary depending on the area measured. For example, capillary pressures are commonly reported as 30–40 mm Hg at the arterial end, 10–14 mm Hg at the venous end, and 25 mm Hg in the middle. Thus, capillary-closing pressures actually range from 12–40 mm Hg. Interface pressures, however, quantify the intensity of pressure being applied externally to the skin, which studies show, commonly exceed capillary pressures.

The general purpose of support surfaces is to reduce these interface pressures by maximizing contact and redistributing weight over a large area. In addition to the pressure reduction or relief that support surfaces provide, many also reduce shear and friction and provide moisture control. Despite the wide range of support-surface products available and the claims of all companies, however, few clinical trials have been conducted. See Figure 2.3 for descriptions and categories of support surfaces.

Specialty mattresses

Everyone has an opinion and personal preferences when it comes to specialty mattresses. These preferences are sometimes based on the product, cost, corporate contracts, or relationship with the sales representative. Clinically, it makes sense that, because pressure ulcer development is based on the intensity and duration of pressure, you need a product that addresses both. For example, a product that solely redistributes pressure (straight low-air loss) to alleviate its intensity does not address the duration component. There are combination products (low-air loss and alternating pressure), however, that can assist with both. Research on some of the three-cell, alternating-pressure surfaces has shown that they increase circulation to the wound and are able to provide pressure elimination in cycles. Some experts, therefore, recommend that you make an alternating pressure component part of the equation.

FIGURE 2.3	**Descriptions/Catagories of Support Surfaces**
Pressure reducing	• Any device that lowers pressure as compared with a standard hospital mattress or chair surface • Do not consistently reduce pressure below capillary closing pressure • Redistributes pressure over a greater area—reducing amounts of pressure at any given point • Almost any product beyond the standard products can legitimately claim pressure reduction—even pool floats (which are not recommended)
Pressure relieving	• Consistently reduce pressure below capillary closing pressure • Conform closely to the patient's body for support and respond to patient's movement • Can be used for prevention of breakdown and to promote healing for a patient with pressure ulcers • Example: Medicare Group 2 powered support surfaces—typically referred to as "specialty beds"
Dynamic	• Surface that decreases tissue interface pressure by altering inflation and deflation • Typically uses electricity to power the inflation/deflation modes • Some specialty beds are "dynamic"
Static	• Reduce pressure by spreading the load over a larger area • Constant inflation is maintained and the surface molds to the body surface • Typically products such as foam, gel, water, or some air overlays
Overlay	• Devices applied over the surface of the mattress • Provide pressure reduction • Increase the height of the bed which may complicate transfers • May be static (foam, gel, water, air filled, low air loss) or dynamic (alternating air)
Replacement mattress	Designed to reduce interface pressures and replaces the typical facility mattress • Usually foam, gel, or air-filled chambers covered with foam • Water-repellent, flame-retardant, antimicrobial top cover • Must have an appropriate indentation load deflection (ILD)
Specialty beds/ low air loss mattress replacements:	• Provide pressure relief by a series of connected air-filled pillows • May have a bed frame or may be a mattress replacement • Amount of pressure can be individualized to provide maximum reduction • Contraindicated for patients with an unstable spine
Specialty beds/ mattress replacements: alternating pressure	• Creates high-pressure and low-pressure areas to prevent constant pressure and to enhance blood flow • Air chambers with air pumped at regular intervals that provide inflation and deflation cycles • Interface pressures lower than capillary closing on deflation and higher when cylinders are inflated
Air fluidized beds	• Helps manage both the intensity and duration of pressure • Contains silicone-coated beads and incorporates fluid and air support • Air pumps through beads and fluidizes the beads • Theoretically "floats" a portion of the body and requires less frequent repositioning • Continuous circulation of warm, dry air may assist with high drainage wounds but may also increase risk of dehydration

When considering whether to use specialty beds, imagine sitting in a soft, overstuffed easy chair. When you first sit down, you are amazingly comfortable, but over a period of time (duration), simple gravity increases the pressure, and you need to reposition yourself to interrupt it. For patients who can't reposition themselves, this pressure an become quite uncomfortable—and, of course, can lead to pressure ulcers.

Understanding foam-mattress characteristics

Standard green-colored hospital mattresses are outdated and associated with high incidences of pressure ulcers. Foam ring "donuts" are also outdated because they concentrate the intensity of the pressure on the surrounding tissue.

Therefore, most hospitals have replaced, or are in the process of replacing, standard mattresses with static pressure-reducing mattresses, most often made of high-density foam. But not all mattresses are created equal. Hospitals spend thousands of dollars each year to purchase foam-replacement mattresses, and too often these decisions are made by cost comparison. Rather, they should be based on knowledge of the characteristics of foam in the context of effective pressure reduction. Such characteristics include base height, density, indentation load deflection (ILD), and contours, defined as follows:

- **Base height** measures foam from its base to where the convolution begins—not to the peak of the convolution. The base height should generally be 4 in.
- **Density,** the weight per cubic foot, measures the amount of foam in the product and reflects its ability to support the patient's weight. Recommended density is 1.3–1.6 pounds per cubic foot.
- **ILD** measures the firmness of foam and is determined by the number of pounds needed to indent it to a depth of 25% of the thickness with a circular plate (e.g., in the case of a 4-in foam mattress, ILD would measure the number of pounds needed to make a 1-in indentation). ILD indicates the ability of the foam to distribute the mechanical load. The goal is to have a low ILD (an ILD of approximately 30 pounds is recommended).
- **ILD ratio,** recommended to be 2.5 or greater, reflects the relationship between conformability and support. A relationship of 60% ILD:25% ILD is needed (e.g., if 30 pounds makes a 1-in depression, then at least 75 pounds would be needed to make a 2.4-in depression in the same foam).
- **Contour** is the surface of the foam, which may be in either slashed, smooth, or egg-crate design. A study by Kemp[2] reported few pressure ulcers when using solid-foam overlay instead of convoluted foam.

In summary, your foam-mattress replacements should include the following features:

- Base height of 4 in
- Density of 1.3–1.6 pounds per cubic foot
- ILD of approximately 30 pounds
- Ratio of 60% ILD to 25% ILD—that is, of 2.5 or greater

"Bottoming out" describes a situation in which the pressure-reducing surface does not provide adequate support. To check for this problem, place a palm up under the mattress or cushion that is below the area at risk of a pressure ulcer. You should feel at least 1 in of support material between your hand and the portion of the "at-risk" skin. If you feel less than 1 in, there is inadequate pressure reduction, and the patient has bottomed out.

Friction and shear

Friction usually, but not always, accompanies shear. Friction is the force of rubbing two surfaces against one another and, friction without force (pressure) causes damage to the epidermis and upper dermal layers and is most commonly known as "sheet burn." Shear is the result of gravity pushing down on the patient's body and the resistance between the patient and the chair or bed. Shear damages the tissue layers that slide against each other and the underlying blood vessels. Therefore, when combined with gravity/force (pressure), friction causes shear, and the outcome can be more devastating then pressure alone.

Observe what happens when the head of the patient's bed is elevated: Gravity pulls the patient's body toward the bottom of the bed, and resistance occurs naturally as the bed tries to hold the body in place. The body isn't held in place, but the skin tries to hold on even as the weight of the body bears down. These circumstances alone are enough to cause damage, but they are compounded in an elderly patient who has dry, inelastic skin and less subcutaneous tissue. Up to 40% of reported pressure ulcers may actually originate from shear.[3]

As a mechanical force perpendicular to an area, pressure alone usually damages the point of impact and the pressure-gradient area discussed earlier. Shear, however, is a parallel mechanical force and therefore damages a wider plane of tissue. Suspect shear forces when the wound is shaped in an irregular pattern (e.g., a triangle), has circumferential undermining, or includes tunneling of sacral ulcers.

Figure 2.4 highlights many of the common practices observed in healthcare facilities that contribute to friction and shear.

| FIGURE 2.4 | Friction and Shear Common Practices |

Common observation or problem	Alternative
Head of bed left elevated (without clinical need to do so)	• Establish an organizationwide practice for managing situations where elevation is maintained for longer than necessary periods. • Example: After meals, incorporate a practice to lower the degree of head elevation when picking up the meal tray or within an hour of the meal—unless clinically contraindicated.
Restless patient that moves feet in bed constantly (friction)	Minimize potential of friction by • placing socks on patient (Note: you may want to use gripper socks in case the patient is someone who may get out of bed alone—to prevent falls associated with stocking feet) • protecting heels with a transparent dressing—alone or in combination with socks • providing heel protectors (preferably seamless) • placing sheepskin at the foot of the bed—although not pressure reducing, it may help reduce friction injury
"Boosting" a patient up in bed	• Use two caregivers and a lift sheet to prevent dragging of the body. • Pay attention to the heels when "boosting" a patient. Even when a lift sheet is used, the heels have a tendency to drag. • Place a pillow under the lower legs to "off-load" the heels, then use the lift sheet to move the patient. Following the boost, the pillow will need to be repositioned. • Ask patient to bend knees and position feet flat on the bed (plantar surface down).
Pulling a brief or incontinence pad from beneath the patient	• Turn patient side-to-side to remove the pad • Under no circumstances should a pad be pulled out from one direction, as doing so will certainly result in skin trauma
Assisting a "maximum assist" patient out of bed alone when two staff are needed	• Always use <u>two</u> people • Lift—don't drag—patient to edge of bed • Resist asking the patient to "scoot" to the edge. The request to "scoot" is usually accompanied by caregiver assistance (force) of the lower extremities, creating a friction/shear force
Dry, inelastic skin	• Moisturizing skin will reduce the incidence of friction injuries
Sliding board transfers	• Carefully inspect skin daily, as sliding creates friction, and the weight of the body provides force • Consider using a trapeze • Consider exiting the bed from alternating sides to minimize repeated forces to the same area of skin
Sagging or sliding down in the chair or wheelchair	• Stand the patient and reseat him/her • Using two caregivers, lift and reposition the patient • Assure proper body alignment and posture • Employ positioning devices identified for the patient

Moisture and incontinence

Urinary incontinence results in overhydration or maceration of the perineal skin. In an overhydrated state, the skin is at greater risk for erosion and impairment of skin integrity. Maceration compromises the skin's ability to function as an effective barrier. Fecal incontinence is even more damaging because of the presence of bacteria and digestive enzymes.

Moisture from incontinence enhances both friction and shear,[4] so it is important to clean and dry the skin promptly after each incontinence episode. If reestablishing continence is possible, initiate a bowel and bladder program. Remember, you reduce the patient's overall risk every time you positively affect a subscale of the risk assessment. Even a change from total incontinence to frequent incontinence positively affects patient risk.

Routine preventive skin care should consist of cleansing, moisturizing, and protection. Learn proper skin cleansing: Avoid vigorous scrubbing, which causes friction and trauma to the skin. Also avoid using typical soap, which changes the skin's acid mantle—a natural antimicrobial—and creates dryness by removing lipids and breaking down fat. Instead, select one of the many incontinence cleaners on the market, preferably one that has a neutral pH and contains moisturizers. Following cleaning, protect the skin with creams or ointments that moisturize the skin and provide a barrier against incontinence.

Seek to establish a hospital protocol for the use of briefs and underpads. Ideally, products should absorb and wick away incontinence moisture from the skin. If your hospital uses cloth briefs, you must change them more frequently because they trap moisture against the skin, which causes maceration. As an alternative to briefs at night or when in bed, an "open system" can prevent the patient from lying on or in a wet cloth. The open system refers to placing an absorbent pad under the patient to wick away moisture. Even when using disposable briefs that wick away moisture, consider using an open system when the patient is in bed because it allows the protection without the risk from snug briefs secured with adhesive tabs.

An open system may be preferable because normal perineal skin, which is slightly acidic pH (5.5), has a tendency to become alkaline when exposed to incontinence. Even moisture caused by perspiration under incontinence briefs can raise the pH (estimated to be 7.1) and increase the risk of dermatitis. Advantages include cost containment, time to air out the skin, and help in maintaining normal skin pH. However, consider the preferences of patients when deciding on which system to use.

Nutritional assessment

Most research relative to nutrition deals with its impact on healing, rather than its role in prevention. Although it has not been definitively determined that improving nutritional intake reduces the incidence of pressure ulcers, various studies and statistics certainly imply that trend. Many studies show that impaired intake is an independent predictor of pressure ulcer development.

Physiologically, it makes sense for malnutrition or protein deficiency to affect the likelihood of pressure ulcer development. If the patient is severely protein deficient, which effects edema formation, his or her soft tissue is more susceptible to breakdown when exposed to pressure. The diffusion of oxygen and nutrients in edematous or ischemic tissue will be compromised. Low protein levels also alter the immune system and result in lower resistance to infection.[5]

Nutrition interventions are important in risk management and must incorporate patient preferences, special needs, and common sense. For instance, medical conditions may require special dietary restrictions, but there may be cases in which the patient chooses not to comply with them. Honor patient preferences within the parameters of those restrictions and note them in the clinical record and care plan as additional risk factors. In addition, allow common sense to prevail in your approaches. Often patients with weight loss and poor dietary intake are provided double portions by staff. But if the patient only consumes 25% of the typical portion, why do we think giving twice as much food will help? In this case, it is better to identify nutrient-dense foods to maximize nutritional and caloric intake.

Also use nutritional assessments to help identify the presence of malnutrition, which often occurs in the elderly. Do not be fooled by the patient's weight: A patient can be overweight and still suffer from malnutrition. Take obesity into account in any event because it also affects mobility, and impaired mobility affects patient risk. Chapter 6 more thoroughly discusses nutritional assessment and laboratory data.

Other factors to consider

Other factors associated with pressure ulcer development include age, body temperature, blood pressure, anemia, hydration, disease, and psychosocial issues. Even in the absence of definitive research, they are all important in your assessment of patient risk.

Age-related changes in skin make it more vulnerable to friction, shear, and pressure. For example, the junction of the dermis and epidermis flattens, making it less resistant to shear forces. This factor makes skin tears more likely in the elderly. In addition, the skin appears thin and transparent due to a decrease in thickness of the dermis. There is also a loss of subcutaneous fat and decreased sensory perception. These changes, along with systemic changes in other body systems, combine to make the skin "at risk."

Increase in body temperature (febrile illness) is also associated with pressure ulcer development. A body-temperature increase is likely related to a combination of decreased activity and the body's struggle to meet the increased oxygen demand, which may shunt it from needy tissue. In addition, dehydration is more likely in this situation and causes increased blood viscosity. Cumulatively, these factors may overwhelm the patient's ability—without support—to prevent pressure ulcers from forming.

Despite the physiology associated with low blood pressure, hypotension is not routinely assessed for its impact on wound development. Postural hypotension is routinely checked for fall risk assessments, for instance, but is never discussed as having an impact with wound development or management—despite the fact that studies[6] show that systolic blood pressures below 100 mm Hg and diastolic pressures below 60 mm Hg are associated with pressure ulcer development. It is also believed that low blood pressure causes blood flow to be shunted to vital organs and away from skin, which may cause lower capillary-closing pressures and therefore make the skin less tolerant of pressure.

What can you do about this problem? Identify hypotension as a risk factor, and work with medical staff to correct it, if possible. Many times, aggressive antihypertensive treatment is so successful that it causes hypotension. From both the fall-risk and pressure ulcer prevention perspectives, it is wise to bring this issue to the attention of medical staff so they can weigh the benefits and risks of the medical care plan. In some cases, for example, hypotension is transient and is related to a fluid deficit, which will reverse when the patient is appropriately hydrated. But you will only know if you ask and assess.

In addition, impaired blood flow to the skin, which can result from many conditions, affects pressure ulcer development and healing. Anemia, for example, results in low erythrocyte (red blood cell) counts. These cells contain hemoglobin, which carries oxygen to the cells, tissues, and organs throughout the body. Other contributors to tissue damage include increased blood viscosity and high hematocrit. In addition, cigarette smoking is cited as a contributing factor in pressure ulcer development because of the physiologic changes that occur with nicotine and the impact on overall oxygenation.

Assess psychosocial status in connection with pressure ulcers. Depression and decreased motivation may affect the patient's overall participation and mobility. In addition, there are chemical changes currently being researched. Psychosocial issues may affect the degree of patients' compliance with interventions and their desire or motivation for avoidance of these complications.

More information on the diseases that affect the likelihood of pressure ulcer development and subsequent healing processes is dispersed throughout the book.

In summary, there are many factors that increase the potential for pressure ulcer development. Systematic assessment is essential in identifying and addressing multiple concomitant factors.

References

1. Agency for Health Care Policy and Research, U.S. Department of Health and Human Services. 1992. Pressure ulcers in adults: Prediction and prevention. AHCPR Publication No. 92-0047. Rockville, MD.

2. Kemp, M.G., et al. 1993. The role of support surfaces and patient attributes in preventing pressure ulcers in elderly patients. *Research in Nursing Health* 16: 89.

3. Bennett, L.M., and B.Y. Lee. 1998. Vertical shear existence in animal pressure threshold experiments. *Decubitus* 1: 18.

4. Ratliff, C.R., and G.T. Redeheaver. 1999. Pressure ulcer assessment and management. *Primary Care Practice* 3: 242–258.

5. Thomas, D.R. 1997. Specific nutritional factors in wound healing. *Advances in Wound Care* 10(4): 40.

6. Bergstrom, N.I. 1997. Strategies for preventing pressure ulcers. *Clinics in Geriatric Medicine* 13(3): 437.

Development and Staging of Pressure Ulcers

Before discussing development and staging of pressure ulcers, we will briefly review skin anatomy and function. This overview is limited to the epidermis, dermis, and subcutaneous tissue (i.e., fat). General knowledge of skin will help you understand the aspects of staging and healing.

Skin anatomy

Skin has the following important characteristics and functions:

- Is the body's largest organ
- Weighs approximately six pounds
- Receives one-third of the body's circulating-blood volume
- Protects against heat, light, injury, and infection
- Regulates body temperature and can sense painful and pleasant stimulation
- Stores water, fat, and vitamin D
- Varies in thickness depending on location, from 0.5 mm in the tympanic membrane
  to 6 mm on the palms of the hands and the soles of the feet

See Figure 3.1 for an illustration of epidermis, dermis, and subcutaneous tissue.

Epidermis

The epidermis is the outermost layer of skin. It is thin, multilayered, avascular (without blood supply), and renewed monthly. The primary function of the epidermis is to provide a protective, waterproof barrier and to resist changes in temperature and pH. The epidermis is almost entirely comprised of keratinocytes, which are important to the skin's function as a protective barrier.

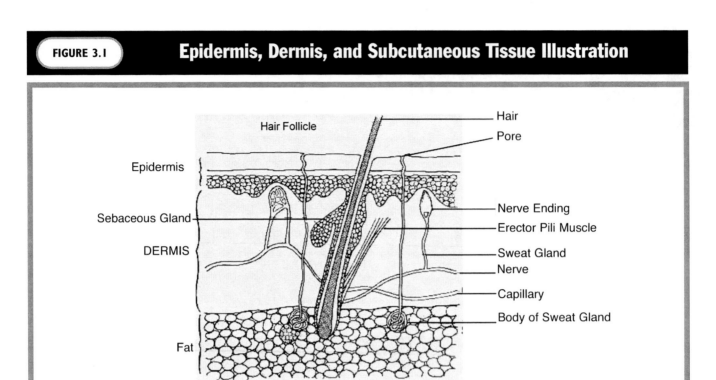

FIGURE 3.1 — **Epidermis, Dermis, and Subcutaneous Tissue Illustration**

Basement membrane

The basement membrane, also known as the epidermal-dermal junction, separates the epidermis from the dermis. It anchors the epidermis to the dermis and is important for elasticity and tensile strength. When a blister forms, this membrane is typically the area that has been damaged.

Dermis

The dermis lies under the epidermis and is the thickest layer of the skin: Its average thickness is 2 mm, or the approximate thickness of a nickel. This layer contains several cell types, including macrophages (known as "scavenger cells"), which ingest bacteria and debris. Mast cells are also found in the dermis; they are important to the inflammatory process and initiate the clotting of blood. The dermis also contains appendages (sweat glands, sebaceous glands), vasculature (capillaries), nerves, and connective tissue (granulation tissue) and provides the structure for the strength of skin.

Subcutaneous tissue

Subcutaneous tissue is the layer of fat below the dermis. It cushions and insulates the body, and it provides support for the dermis and epidermis. It also works as a shock absorber to help protect other organs from injury and is basically a reserve tank for energy (yes, that is where the extra calories are stored!).

Skin must be safeguarded so it can undergo its normal functions of sensation, protection, thermoregulation, communication, and metabolism. Aging skin is already compromised due to physiologic changes—fibroblasts are less efficient, collagen synthesis wanes, and the thickness and elasticity of the dermis decreases—which heightens the need for careful skin care and preventive practices. But other age-related changes affect pressure ulcer prevention and wound healing:

- The basement membrane (epidermal-dermal junction) flattens, which makes it more susceptible to friction and shear.

- The ability to repair tissue decreases.

- Collagen deposits decline, resulting in less skin elasticity.

- The turnover of epidermal cells takes longer.

- Sensation decreases.

- Macrophages and sebaceous glands slow down, which results in delayed cleaning and repair of the wound. This is an important change for wound healing. Think of machrophage function as taking out the garbage: The more you delay, the more garbage accumulates, and this "pile-up" slows down your housekeeping. Likewise, inefficient macrophages delay the ultimate rate of wound healing.

With all of the physiological changes that occur with aging, prevention takes on even greater importance.

Staging of pressure ulcers

The staging of pressure ulcers depicts tissue damage related to pressure. The same basic staging criteria have been in place for more than 10 years, but many nurses do not consistently follow proper staging. Information about pressure ulcers is covered only superficially, if at all, in today's standard nursing education programs. Therefore, student nurses are not being trained to conduct thorough assessments of a condition affecting millions of people across the country. To compound the problem, many healthcare settings have limited support and education for new nurses to develop this skill post-graduation. These circumstances lead to incomplete and often inaccurate assessments—and ultimately pose a risk-management dilemma.

Pressure ulcers are staged using a universal system from the Wound, Ostomy and Continence Nurse (WOCN) Society in 1992 and the National Pressure Ulcer Advisory Panel (NPUAP) in 1999. Each stage reflects the type and depth of observed damage. Staging is intended to show tissue destruction, not healing. The following describes the four stages of pressure ulcers (key staging criteria are bolded for emphasis):

Note: Please refer to your laminated sheet to review photographs (#1–6) of pressure ulcers Stages I–IV.

Stage I: An observable, pressure-related alteration of intact skin, whose indicators, as compared with the adjacent or opposite area on the body, may include changes in one or more of the following:

- Skin temperature (e.g., coolness or warmth)
- Tissue consistency (e.g., firm or boggy)
- Sensation (e.g., pain or itching)

The ulcer appears as a defined area of persistent redness in lightly pigmented skin, whereas in darker skin, the ulcer may appear with red, blue, or purple hues.

Stage II: A **partial-thickness skin** loss involving the epidermis, dermis, or both. The ulcer presents clinically as an abrasion, a blister, or a shallow crater.

Stage III: Full-thickness skin loss involving damage or necrosis of subcutaneous tissue, which may extend down to but not through underlying fascia. The ulcer presents clinically as a deep crater, with or without undermining of adjacent tissue.

Stage IV: Full-thickness skin loss with extensive destruction, tissue necrosis, or damage to muscle, bone, or supporting structures such as tendon or joint capsule.

Documentation changes

If a patient's Stage IV ulcer improves, document it as a "healing Stage IV." Validate your opinion by documenting characteristics of the wound such as width, depth, presence or absence of necrotic tissue, exudate, and presence of granulation tissue. Always be descriptive and avoid using statements such as "healing slowly" or "healing well."

Remember, the staging classification system is only meant to depict tissue damage related to pressure, not to classify all wounds.

How do you classify non-pressure–related skin breakdown?

Wagner Grading System

Numerous classification scales are available for non-pressure–related wounds. One such scale is the Wagner Grading System for vascular wounds on the extremities. The Wagner Grading System provides a numerical grade and characteristics of that grade (see Figure 3.2).

FIGURE 3.2	Wagner Grading System
Grade	**Characteristics**
0	• Pre-ulcerative lesion • Healed ulcers • Presence of bony deformity
1	Superficial ulcer without subcutaneous involvement
2	Ulcer with penetration through the subcutaneous tissue (that may expose bone, tendon, ligament, joint capsule)
3	Ulcer with penetration through the subcutaneous tissue (that may expose bone, tendon, ligament, joint capsule)
4	Gangrene of a digit
5	Gangrene of the foot requiring disarticulation

Partial thickness and full thickness

The terms partial and full thickness reflect the amount of damaged skin tissue. Partial-thickness wounds are confined to the epidermal layer and may include, but do not penetrate beyond, the dermis. Full thickness indicates damage of the epidermis, dermis, and subcutaneous tissue or beyond. These terms cannot stand alone and must be incorporated into your typical assessment of the wound (e.g., type of tissue observed, depth of wound).

If you compare the staging terminology to the definitions of partial thickness and full thickness, you will notice they share definitions. For instance, partial thickness is the equivalent to Stage II pressure ulcer destruction. The same goes for full thickness, which is the equivalent to a Stage III/IV pressure ulcer.

It is important that you understand the difference in terminology, because if you classify non-pressure–related ulcers using pressure ulcer staging, others may conclude that they are pressure areas. There is a tendency for nurses (and physicians) to refer to all tissue damage as pressure ulcers and to stage the wound. This inaccuracy is troubling from the perspectives of treatment, regulations, and risk management. Remember: You cannot classify all extremity wounds as partial thickness or full thickness. If the origin is pressure, it should be staged; if the origin is not pressure, use other scales or descriptors.

The NPUAP position statement and reverse staging

A NPUAP position statement titled "The Facts about Reverse Staging in 2000—The NPUAP Position Statement" thoroughly outlined the problem with backstaging (i.e., reverse staging). See the NPUAP Web site at *www.npuap.org/positn5.html* for the text of the position statement.

The NPUAP makes a strong, clinically based case *against* reverse staging.

Why backstaging doesn't work

Backstaging does not work because a site of a healed pressure ulcer always represents an area of weakness in skin integrity. Even after the area is closed and has an opportunity to remodel (which could take up to two years), it will only have approximately 75% of the tensile strength of undamaged skin. It may eventually look the same as the remaining tissue, but it will never be the same again. Granulation tissue is just scar tissue. This is the main reason that backstaging is clinically inappropriate: It implies that there is a replacement of normal tissue components as it heals, which simply isn't the case.

Healing processes for Stage IIs v. Stage III/IVs

Stage III and Stage IV pressure ulcers heal by filling with granulation tissue and then re-epithelializing. On the other hand, Stage II pressure ulcers only re-epithelialize. The healing process for a Stage II is more efficient and less complicated.

What is the relevance to your practice? Wound assessment and descriptions in the patient's progress or treatment notes often indicate that a healing Stage II pressure ulcer has granulation tissue. But if there granulation tissue exists in the wound, then it was not a Stage II, and its true depth may have been incorrectly staged. If the body required the assistance of granulation tissue to fill the defect, then the pressure ulcer was at least a Stage III/IV.

This physiologic fact is also important to incorporate into your clinical thinking and assessment of patients admitted with pressure ulcers. If another healthcare facility sends you a patient, and the transfer paperwork reflects a Stage II pressure ulcer, but you also observe granulation tissue in the initial wound assessment, proceed with caution. In this case, you can document the disparity and the rationale for your assessment. Even though you don't know the history of the wound, your assessment should be accurate. You may need to document the wound as a Stage II based on the current appearance and the unknown history. From a clinically accurate and risk-management point of view, your complete assessment is valuable.

Wound healing

Significant research is being conducted on the various roles of growth factors, including cytokines, proteases, and extracellular matrix molecules, just to name a few. The purpose of this book isn't to overwhelm the reader with molecular biology, but knowledgeable wound care requires at least a basic understanding of the phases of wound healing. Subsequent chapters deal with assessment and treatment; therefore, you need to understand what you can expect to see and what constitutes a deviation from the norm. In a perfect world, wounds would progress in an orderly fashion through the three stages, but they do not.

There are three general phases of wound healing:

1. Inflammatory phase
2. Proliferative phase
3. Maturation phase

Inflammatory phase

The inflammatory phase begins moments after injury and lasts approximately three days post-injury. The primary objective of this phase is to control the bleeding, clean up debris and bacteria, and prevent infection. Moments after the wound occurs, vasoconstriction allows the area to clot and provides the initial release of growth factors to attract inflammatory cells—the body's way of summoning help. The blood vessels dilate to allow fluid and cells into the "scene" of the accident. Neutrophils, some of the first responders, then begin removing bacteria and debris.

Inflammation gets a lot of bad publicity, but it is both expected and helpful in this phase of wound healing. Inflammation communicates the need for additional materials required to heal the wound. See Figure 3.3 for examples of the types of cells and their functions during this process.

FIGURE 3.3	**Cells and Their Functions During Inflammation**

Polymorphonucler cells and monocytes	• Turn into macrophages for clean up of the wound
Macrophages	• If in the presence of adequate Vitamin A, release growth factors and attract fibroblasts and lymphocytes
Fibroblasts and lymphocytes	• Release cytokines (additional growth factors)
Cytokines	• Needed in adequate amounts in the inflammatory phase and subsequent phases

The inflammatory phase should last only a few days. It is not normal for signs of inflammation to remain a week or more after injury. Many chronic wounds get stuck in the inflammatory phase, which causes delays in the healing process and leads to an overabundance of proteases (i.e., enzymes) that break down tissue. Two such proteases, elastase and matrix metalloproteinase (MMP-8), destroy growth factors and the foundation of the wound.

Relevance to practice

• Prolonged inflammation is too much of a good thing: It actually becomes damaging due to the presence of too many proteases. Regular debridement of the wound will decrease proteases and will facilitate progression into the proliferative phase.

Proliferative phase

This phase lasts approximately three to 21 days after completion of the inflammatory phase. In reality, the phases often overlap and sometimes "yo-yo" back and forth between inflammation and proliferation, especially if the bacterial burden is increasing. That is one reason why revisiting debridement is sometimes necessary.

Ideally, this is a growth phase. New connective tissue, comprised of fibroblasts, collagen fibers, and new blood vessels, fills the wound. The job description of this phase includes synthesis of collagen, release of growth factors, formation of new blood vessels, formation of granulation tissue to fill the wound defect, wound contraction, and epithelialization.

Wound contraction is the pulling together of the wound edges. This process occurs as fibroblasts "morph" into myofibroblasts, which have contractile abilities. Epithelialization is the migration and proliferation of epithelial cells from the wound edges and will ultimately resurface the wound. Epithelial tissue is very fragile, pink, and usually present at the wound edges initially and in small areas throughout the wound. Epithelial cells travel across the open wound bed, facilitated by moisture and guided by collagen in the underlying wound.

Relevance to practice

- The wound tissue formed during this phase is granulation tissue. It appears beefy red and bumpy (granular). It most resembles the side of a strawberry. (If the wound is pale and the tissue has edema, there may be an infection even if not accompanied by erythema or purulence.)

- The defect fills with the granulation tissue: It covers with new epithelium, but a new dermal layer is not a part of the repair.

Maturation phase

The maturation phase begins approximately 21 days after injury and may take years to finish. In this phase, the collagen rearranges (i.e., remodels) to maximize the strength of the tissue. Collagen is the major component of scar tissue. Fibroblasts decline in number, vascularity decreases, and tensile strength begins to improve. Resurfaced wounds may regain 50% of their original tensile strength three weeks post-injury, but no matter what the subsequent passage of time, it will only achieve a maximum of 75% of its original strength.

Relevance to practice

- When you have finally succeeded in closing a wound, remember to educate the patient and family members that it will be a continuing struggle to prevent recurrence of a pressure ulcer in that area.

Assessing risk and establishing preventive strategies are the most critical aspects of pressure ulcer prevention. Despite their importance, however, they often are denied critical thought and integration in the immediate plan of care for the patient. Determining a patient's risk-assessment score is an informative process, but unless nurses identify the risk factors that contributed to the score—and minimize those deficits—doing so is pointless.

Nurses are commonly able to recite the risk-assessment schedule but unable to answer the question, "Now that you have assessed the patient to be high risk, what do you do?" Nurses need to know automatically what steps to put in place immediately upon identification of a high-risk patient. They need to have access to effective policies and procedures, supplies for pressure relief and skin protection, and a clear understanding of their responsibility to act contemporaneously wiith their indentification of a high-risk patient.

Risk-assessment tools

The most widely used risk-assessment tools are the Braden Scale and the Norton Scale. These scales query subsets of information that are assigned numerical ratings, which ultimately determine a patient's risk score/level. Clinical research supports the reliability and validity of both scales.

The Braden Scale has six subscales that correspond to our prior discussion of intensity and duration of pressure and tissue tolerance for pressure (see Figure 4.1). Three subscales—sensory perception, mobility, and activity—address factors that expose the patient to intensity and duration of pressure. The remaining three—moisture, nutrition, and friction/shear—address factors that affect tissue tolerance. Each subscale is ranked numerically, and the subscale scores are totaled to provide a final score. Total scores can range from six to 23, and as the scores become lower, predicted risk rises.

| FIGURE 4.1 | **Braden Scale for Predicting Pressure Sore Risk** |

Patient's Name _____ Evaluator's Name _____ Date of Assessment _____

Category	1	2	3	4
SENSORY PERCEPTION ability to respond meaningfully to pressure-related discomfort	**1. Completely Limited** Unresponsive (does not moan, flinch, or grasp) to painful stimuli, due to diminished level of con-sciousness or sedation. OR limited ability to feel pain over most of body	**2. Very Limited** Responds only to painful stimuli. Cannot communicate discomfort except by moaning or restlessness OR has a sensory impairment which limits the ability to feel pain or discomfort over ½ of body.	**3. Slightly Limited** Responds to verbal com-mands, but cannot always communicate discomfort or the need to be turned. OR has some sensory impairment which limits ability to feel pain or discomfort in 1 or 2 extremities.	**4. No Impairment** Responds to verbal commands. Has no sensory deficit which would limit ability to feel or voice pain or discomfort..
MOISTURE degree to which skin is exposed to moisture	**1. Constantly Moist** Skin is kept moist almost constantly by perspiration, urine, etc. Dampness is detected every time patient is moved or turned.	**2. Very Moist** Skin is often, but not always moist. Linen must be changed at least once a shift.	**3. Occasionally Moist:** Skin is occasionally moist, requiring an extra linen change approximately once a day.	**4. Rarely Moist** Skin is usually dry, linen only requires changing at routine intervals.
ACTIVITY degree of physical activity	**1. Bedfast** Confined to bed.	**2. Chairfast** Ability to walk severely limited or non-existent. Cannot bear own weight and/or must be assisted into chair or wheelchair.	**3. Walks Occasionally** Walks occasionally during day, but for very short distances, with or without assistance. Spends majority of each shift in bed or chair	**4. Walks Frequently** Walks outside room at least twice a day and inside room at least once every two hours during waking hours
MOBILITY ability to change and control body position	**1. Completely Immobile** Does not make even slight changes in body or extremity position without assistance	**2. Very Limited** Makes occasional slight changes in body or extremity position but unable to make frequent or significant changes independently.	**3. Slightly Limited** Makes frequent though slight changes in body or extremity position independently.	**4. No Limitation** Makes major and frequent changes in position without assistance.
NUTRITION usual food intake pattern	**1. Very Poor** Never eats a complete meal. Rarely eats more than ⅓ of any food offered. Eats 2 servings or less of protein (meat or dairy products) per day. Takes fluids poorly. Does not take a liquid dietary supplement OR is NPO and/or maintained on clear liquids or IV's for more than 5 days.	**2. Probably Inadequate** Rarely eats a complete meal and generally eats only about ½ of any food offered. Protein intake includes only 3 servings of meat or dairy products per day. Occasionally will take a dietary supplement OR receives less than optimum amount of liquid diet or tube feeding	**3. Adequate** Eats over half of most meals. Eats a total of 4 servings of protein (meat, dairy products per day. Occasionally will refuse a meal, but will usually take a supplement when offered OR is on a tube feeding or TPN regimen which probably meets most of nutritional needs	**4. Excellent** Eats most of every meal. Never refuses a meal. Usually eats a total of 4 or more servings of meat and dairy products. Occasionally eats between meals. Does not require supplementation.
FRICTION & SHEAR	**1. Problem** Requires moderate to maximum assistance in moving. Complete lifting without sliding against sheets is impossible. Frequently slides down in bed or chair, requiring frequent repositioning with maximum assistance. Spasticity, contractures or agitation leads to almost constant friction	**2. Potential Problem** Moves feebly or requires minimum assistance. During a move skin probably slides to some extent against sheets, chair, restraints or other devices. Maintains relatively good position in chair or bed most of the time but occasionally slides down.	**3. No Apparent Problem** Moves in bed and in chair independently and has sufficient muscle strength to lift up completely during move. Maintains good position in bed or chair.	

Total Score _____

Source: Used with permission. © Copyright Barbara Braden and Nancy Bergstrom, 1988   All rights reserved

The Norton Scale has five subscales—physical condition, mental condition, activity, mobility, and incontinence (see Figure 4.2). Each subscale has a numerical ranking, and total scores can range from five to 20. There is also a Norton Plus Scale that includes additional point deductions for diagnosis of diabetes or hypertension, low hemoglobin and hematocrit, low albumin level, febrile illness, five or more medications, and changes in mental status over the past 24 hours.

Although both the Braden and Norton scales are the validated tools for risk assessment, they assess patient risk factors differently than each other. For example, with the Braden scale, the following risk factors are assessed:

- Sensory perception
- Moisture
- Friction and shear
- Nutrition

With the Norton scale, the following risk factors are assessed:

- Incontinence
- Physical condition
- Mental condition

Both scales assess activity and mobility.

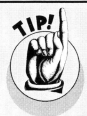

Documentation tip

Remember to practice accurate documentation practices of all risk assessments to ensure continuity of care and to use as a foundation for the patient's skin care plan.

Numerous intrinsic and extrinsic factors play a role in overall risk. Even if the particular scale used does not measure other risk factors, include them in your critical-thinking process. Researchers[1] have identified other risk factors that include low diastolic pressure (less than 60), ages over 80 years, poor current dietary protein intake, vascular disease, and pain. Pain is an important factor that often reveals itself as immobility or under-nutrition. Chapter 6 more thoroughly reviews pain as a factor. See Figure 4.3 for a chart of intrinsic and extrinsic factors.

FIGURE 4.2 — Norton Scale

Norton Scale

NOTE: Scores of 14 or less rate the patient as 'at risk'

Name	Date	Physical Condition				Mental Condition				Activity				Mobility				Incontinence				Total Score
		Good	4			Alert	4			Ambulant	4			Full	4			Not	4			
		Fair	3			Apathetic	3			Walk-help	3			Slightly limited	3			Occasional	3			
		Poor	2			Confused	2			Chair-bound	2			Very limited	2			Usually/urine	2			
		Very bad	1			Stupor	1			Bedridden	1			Immobile	1			Doubly	1			

Source: Doreen Norton, Rhoda McLaren and A N Exton-Smith, *An Investigation of Geriatric Nursing Problems in Hospital 8, National Corporation for the Care of Old People (now Centre for Policy on Ageing), London, 1962.*

FIGURE 4.3 — Chart of Intrinsic and Extrinsic Factors

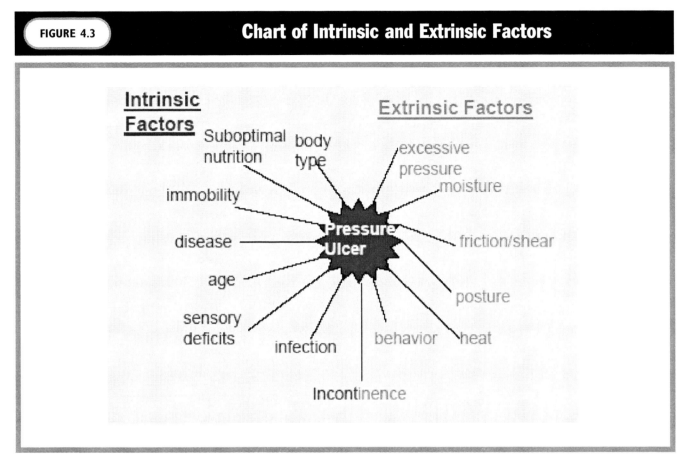

No matter which scale you use, what's important is the action you take as a result of the scores within the context of the total assessment of the patient. See Figure 4.4 for an example of scoring using both scales. At each level of risk, when viewed in the context of the patient's overall health and functional status, you may need to be more aggressive with prevention activities.

FIGURE 4.4 — Scoring Using Braden and Norton Scales

	Mild risk	Moderate risk	High risk	Very high risk
Braden Scale	15–18	13–14	10–12	9 or below
Norton Scale	14	13	12	—

As a nurse, you must determine the purpose of conducting an assessment and your follow-up responsibilities. Nursing management should convey the following to you:

- Expectations of conducting the risk assessment, which include identifying who is responsible for the first assessment and establishing a deadline for that assessment
- Hospital protocol for high-risk patients
- Location of the supplies
- Identification of who has access to supplies
- A permanent method of informing nursing assistants, or nursing technicians, of their responsibilities in providing care to patients with pressure ulcers (e.g., repositioning the patient, using incontinence products, and providing pressure-relief wheelchair cushions)

If you wait for the comprehensive assessment that occurs two weeks after admission instead of starting pressure ulcer prevention care right away, you will have failed to protect patients during their most vulnerable period.

Frequency of risk assessment

In acute care, pressure ulcers usually develop within the first two weeks of hospitalization.[2] The Agency for Healthcare Research and Quality Guidelines state that "active, mobile individuals should be reassessed for changes in activity and mobility status. The frequency of reassessment depends on patient status and institutional policy. The condition of an individual admitted to a healthcare facility is not static; consequently, pressure ulcer risk requires routine re-examination." In their article, "How and Why to Do Pressure Ulcer Risk Assessments," Braden and Ayello recommend initial assessment on admission, then reassessment at least every 48 hours or whenever the patient's condition changes.[3]

Risk-assessment tools are adjuncts to your clinical judgment. Intrinsic and extrinsic risk factors and the patient's clinical presentation form the basis for the prevention program.

Areas of highest risk for pressure ulcer development

The areas of highest risk for pressure ulcer development depend on the physical positioning of the patient. When the patient is seated, the ischial tuberosity is exposed to the highest risk, but when the patient is lying down, the sacrum is at the highest risk. The location of the pressure ulcer will often indicate its origin. See Figure 4.5 for a diagram of pressure points.

FIGURE 4.5 **Pressure Points**

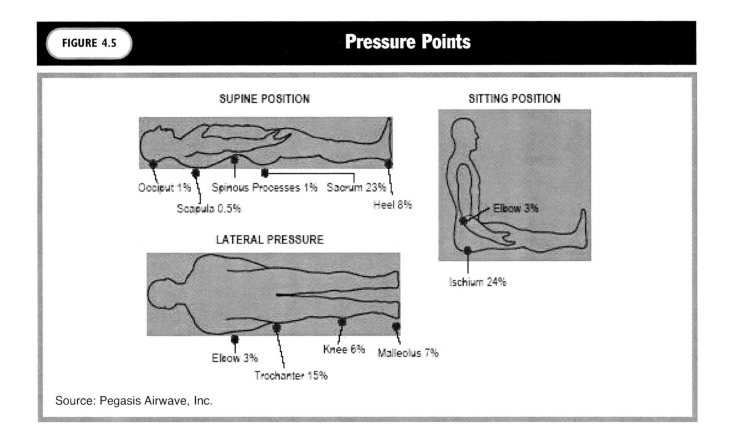

SUPINE POSITION

Occiput 1% | Spinous Processes 1% | Sacrum 23%

Scapula 0.5% | Heel 8%

LATERAL PRESSURE

Elbow 3% | Knee 6% | Malleolus 7%

Trochanter 15%

SITTING POSITION

Elbow 3%

Ischium 24%

Source: Pegasis Airwave, Inc.

References

1. Bergstrom, N., and B. Braden. 1992. A prospective study of pressure sore risk among institutionalized elderly. *Journal of the American Geriatrics Society* 40: 747–58.

2. Langemo, D.K., B. Olson, S. Hunter, C. Burd, D. Hansen, and T. Cathcart-Silberberg. 1989. Incidence of pressure sores in acute care, rehabilitation, extended care, home health, and hospice in one locale. *Decubitus* 2(2): 42.

3. Braden, B., and A. Ayello. 2002. How and Why to Do Pressure Ulcer Risk Assessments? *Advances in Skin & Wound Care* 15(3): 125–131.

Wound Assessment

Assessment forms the basis for treating the whole patient, not just the "hole" in the patient. Thorough assessment is the foundation for developing a comprehensive treatment plan and modifying that plan on an ongoing basis. Unfortunately, there are still many medical and nursing staff who believe that wound assessment is limited to a weekly measurement of the wound. Accepted standards of practice require a comprehensive assessment of the pressure ulcer on admission and reassessment at least weekly to ensure the wound is progressing toward healing. In her book *Acute and Chronic Wounds*, Ruth Bryant suggests, for patients who need more frequent dressing changes, that "acute-care wound assessments . . . be documented with every dressing change but not to exceed once per day." This chapter details the components of a comprehensive assessment, including macroscopic wound indices that should be assessed.

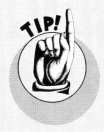

Documentation tip

It is important to know the correct terminology as it relates to pressure ulcers and their care. You will need to use such terms when completing the documentation that comes with assessing and reassessing patients' plans of care.

Types of tissue

There are four types of tissue to observe in a pressure ulcer: *epithelial, granulation, slough,* and *eschar/necrosis.* Epithelial and granulation tissue are viable (living), and slough and eschar tissues are nonviable (nonliving). All four types of tissue can be present in one pressure ulcer.

Epithelial tissue is fragile, pink tissue that forms in the process of healing. In a Stage II pressure ulcer, this tissue may be observed not only at the edges but also throughout the bed of the wound. The epithelial cells migrate across a moist wound surface. In a Stage III or Stage IV, however, epithelial tissue will be observed only at the edges of the pressure ulcer. The tissue is typically pale pink and translucent-appearing because epithelial tissue is avascular.

Granulation tissue is typically red and moist and often is described by the term "beefy red." This tissue contains new blood vessels and connective tissue. Granulation tissue fills the cavity of deeper wounds and is only observed in Stage III or Stage IV pressure ulcers or full-thickness wounds. With its velvety, granular appearance, healthy granulation tissue looks like the side of a strawberry. It may also appear as pale pink or dull red in deep wounds that have a suboptimal vascular supply.

An accumulation of dead cellular debris, **slough** is dead tissue in the process of separating from viable tissue. It is usually yellow or yellowish white due to the large number of leukocytes present. Be careful when assessing this tissue because other tissue, including subcutaneous tissue or tendons, may also have this color. Although slough can give you an idea of the level of tissue destruction, you cannot stage the wound when it is present. Figure 5.1 describes various stages of slough.

FIGURE 5.1	Various Stages of Slough
Stringy, yellow slough	May indicate that subcutaneous fat tissue has died
Thicker, yellow slough	May indicate muscle degeneration
Hard, black eschar	Indicates full-thickness destruction

Documenting characteristics of slough provides a more comprehensive pressure ulcer assessment because not all slough is created equal. The term is not all-encompassing and, depending on other descriptors, may alter your treatment approach. The descriptors in Figure 5.2 may be used for nonviable tissue wound documentation.

Non-adherent yellow slough	Thin, mucous-like material that separates easily from wound tissue
Loosely adherent yellow slough	Thick, stringy material that often appears as a clump of debris that is attached to wound tissue
Soft adherent black eschar	Soggy (mushy) tissue that is firmly attached to tissue in the center of the wound or the base of the wound
Firmly adherent, hard black eschar	Crusty, firm tissue that is strongly attached to the base/edges of the wound

FIGURE 5.2 — **Descriptors for Non-Viable–Tissue Documentation**

Eschar is dead tissue that is thick, black, and leathery. Although eschar can be soft and adherent, most often it is firm and hard. Eschar is a type of necrotic tissue, as is slough. Nurses often document necrosis as an interchangeable term with eschar, but remember that necrosis is dead tissue that could be slough or eschar. If you document necrotic tissue, further describe it as slough or eschar. Note: *Please refer to your laminated sheet to review photograph #7, Heel with eschar.*

As previously stated, you may observe more than one tissue type in a wound. Note the percentage of each tissue type because typically, treatment decisions are based in part on the predominant tissue type. For example, if a pressure ulcer is 75% slough and 25% granulation tissue, the highest priority would be debridement. If percentages are reversed, however, and granulation tissue is predominant, then the treatment goal should include maintaining a moist wound environment and protection of the granulation tissue.

Exudate type and amount

Exudate is the fluid accumulated in the wound. This drainage fluid is composed of leukocytes, bacteria, serum, natural-growth factors, and cell debris and is often helpful in wound healing. Therefore, aggressive washing or drying of new wounds may harm them both by interfering with the natural contributions exudate makes and by removing the moist environment needed to promote wound healing. Certainly you are interested in washing out or diluting dead tissue and bacteria, but recognize that you also affect the protein and nutrients present in serum and growth factors. One positive aspect of dressings with extended wearing time is that they may allow the body's own fluid to bathe the wound. *Note: Please refer to your laminated sheet to review photograph #8, Exudate.*

Note the type of exudate with every dressing change. Avoid dressings that produce a gel or that "melt" into the wound, as they make it difficult to assess the type of exudate. After dressing removal, cleanse the wound and then assess for the type of drainage. There may be more than one, and in that instance, note both and document the predominant type (see Figure 5.3).

FIGURE 5.3 — **Types of Exudates Drainage**

Serous	• Clear or straw colored
	• Thin and watery
Serosanguinous	• Slightly bloody drainage with serous characteristics
	• Thin, watery. May be pink or pale red
Sanguinous	• Bloody, thin, bright red drainage
Purulent	• Thick, opaque drainage
	• Tan or yellow appearance
	• A product of inflammation that contains pus—contains leukocytes, bacteria, and cell debris
Foul purulent	• Thick, opaque drainage
	• Yellow or green or in the spectrum between)
	• A product of inflammation that contains pus—contains leukocytes, bacteria, and cell debris
	• Offensive odor

Also note the *amount of exudate*. There is great variation in the reporting of the wound exudate. Because it is impractical to measure the drainage that soaks through the dressings, you are left with less precise methods of quantifying drainage. Most hospitals quantify drainage with terms such as *none, scant, small, moderate,* and *large* (or *copious*) (see Figure 5.4). Remember that assessment of wound exudate is not entirely dependent on the dressing, and it also must include assessment of the wound tissues.

FIGURE 5.4	**Definitions of Drainage Terms**

None	• Dressing is dry • Wound tissue is dry
Scant	• Wound tissue is moist • No quantifiable exudates
Small	• Wound tissue is wet and there is moisture throughout the wound • Drainage is apparent on less than 25% of the dressing
Moderate	• Wound tissues are saturated • Drainage may be distributed throughout the wound or may be pooled is certain areas of the wound • Drainage is apparent on 25%–75% of the dressing
Large/Copious	• Wound tissues are saturated • Drainage is seeping/rolling out of the wound • Drainage may be distributed throughout the wound or may be pooled in certain areas • Drainage is apparent on more than 75% of the dressing

Odor

Most wounds have an odor that can be detected at dressing changes. Odor can be associated with certain categories of dressings and also may be due to poor containment of wound drainage or insufficient frequency of dressing change. Therefore, it is important to remove the dressing and clean the wound before determining that a foul odor exists. If the wound has a strong odor, that odor will remain after wound cleansing. Such foul odor often signifies the presence of anaerobic organisms. Fruity odors are often associated with *staphylococcus* organisms; fecal-like odors are often associated with gram-negative bacteria. If you suspect that the pressure ulcer is infected based on the odor or other characteristics, notify a physician. According to the Agency for Healthcare Research and Quality guidelines, bacteremia and sepsis associated with pressure ulcers are commonly caused by *Staphylococcus aureus*, gram-negative rods, or *Bacteroides fragilis*. If a patient develops clinical signs of sepsis (i.e., fever, tachycardia, hypotension, decreased mental status), seek immediate medical attention.

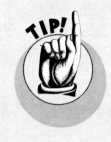

Patient care tip

To help reduce the patient's anxiety about offensive wound odor, consider dressing the wound with charcoal properties or other commercial products that decrease odor.

Undermining and sinus tracts

In your assessment, evaluate the presence of undermining or sinus tracts. Conduct the assessment by gently probing the wound bed with a cotton-tipped applicator. If you prefer, supplement this inspection with external peri-wound palpation (sometimes sinus tracts can be detected externally).

Undermining

Undermining is a space under the surface of the skin that only is open at the skin surface. It is closed at the interior aspect of the wound and presents like a free edge or shelf of skin. Undermining usually involves a larger area of the wound edge. Most often, it appears as a result of subcutaneous-fat death, and it usually is associated with pressure ulcers that are suffering additional trauma from shear forces. Less frequently, undermining is associated with anaerobic organisms.

When assessing undermining, measure both the extent of undermining (parallel to the wound) and the amount of wound edge involved. Measure depth in centimeters and describe the location of the undermining using the face of a clock (i.e., 12:00 would be toward the patient's head). Undermining can occur on all edges of the wound.

Sinus tract or tunnel

A sinus tract or tunnel is a channel underlying a wound of which there can be more than one. It typically has a smaller edge than undermining and extends in only one direction. A sinus tract results in dead space and has a potential for abscess formation, so locating and measuring it is essential. As when measuring undermining, use a cotton-tipped applicator to gently probe, find the opening of the tract, and slowly advance until resistance is felt. Measure the depth at this point. Wound documentation should indicate the location of the sinus tract(s) using the face of the clock, the direction of the tract, and the measurement in centimeters.

Wound edge

A wound edge is another key component of pressure ulcer assessment that is often neglected. It is surprising how little attention it is given—a closed or hyperkeratotic wound edge indicates a nonhealing wound and so should be monitored. The most common descriptors for wound edges include closed *(epibole)*, open, *hyperkeratotic*, and *macerated* (see Figure 5.5). Other descriptions include evaluation of the attachment of the wound edge.

FIGURE 5.5	**Common Descriptors for Wound Edges**
Closed wound edge	• Top layers of the epidermis roll down and cover lower edge of epidermis, which prevents epithelial cell migration • Also called epibole • Appears hard, thick, and rolled
Hyperkeratotic edge	• Hard, white-gray tissue • Appears callus-like
Macerated edge	• Softening of tissue from over-exposure to fluids (wound drainage, wet dressings) • Appears like "dish pan" hands
Open edge	• Edge is healthy—usually flesh colored and often with evidence of new tissue growth at the rim

Remember that a pressure ulcer with a closed edge will not heal until the edge is reopened. Often nurses change the treatment of the wound numerous times due to delayed wound closure, even when the problem is not the treatment but rather the closed wound edge. In the case of epibole, or closed wound edges, surgical debridement or chemical cauterization (with silver nitrate sticks) by medical staff is generally necessary.

Peri-wound appearance

Assess the condition of the skin around a pressure ulcer. There is a tendency to be myopic when assessing wounds, so if you "can't see the forest for the trees," step back and observe the whole picture. The peri-wound condition must be part of this assessment. Think back to wound assessments in which the initial pressure ulcer is making positive progress but numerous other open areas have occurred in a windowpane configuration from the dressing adhesives.

Therefore, make peri-wound assessment a priority. Assess for erythema, edema, induration, warmth, crepitus, and other signs of infection. Is the skin macerated? Rashy? Discolored? Then look for damage from previous dressings or from tape and adhesives. When the skin around the pressure ulcer is fragile, excoriated, erythematous, or edematous, the size and placement of the dressing likely needs to be altered. Such alteration sometimes will result in a dressing that is disproportionate to the size of the pressure ulcer, but such incongruity is necessary to give relief to the affected peri-wound skin.

Measuring pressure ulcers

Wound measurement is the most-often conducted aspect of pressure ulcer assessment, although there is wide variability in technique. Measurements are an important parameter when reviewed in the context of a *complete* assessment. In 1883, Lord Kelvin, the British scientist who laid the foundation for modern physics and the absolute-temperature scale named for him, said, "When you can measure what you are speaking about and express it in numbers, you know something about it; but when you cannot measure it, when you cannot express it in numbers, your knowledge is of a meager and unsatisfactory kind; it may be the beginning of knowledge, but you have scarcely in your thoughts advanced to the state of science, whatever the matter may be."

Wound measurement helps determine wound status. It may alert the nurse and physician to a need for changes in treatment strategy. It is an objective parameter that provides a basis for clinical decision-making when used in the context of the complete assessment. Additionally, wound measurement is an important factor in risk management. The expected and accepted standard of practice (against which you are measured) is complete documentation of wound size and characteristics. Pressure ulcer litigation generally relies on deviations from accepted standards of care, and measurement is one basic standard that is *always* evaluated.

Wounds can be measured in a variety of ways, and a brief review of techniques follow. A thorough discussion of linear measurements is provided because this is the measurement technique most often used. Wound measurement is either **two-dimensional** (length x width) or **three-dimensional** (length x width x depth).

FIGURE 5.6	**Two-Dimensional Measurement Techniques**
Planimetry	• Complete graph squares within a wound tracing or photograph are counted • Can be useful for irregularly shaped or large wounds and is best suited to flat wounds • Area calculated in planimetry is documented as square centimeters (cm2) • Counting squares manually is inefficient—researchers using computer technology more apt to use this than nurses
Stereophotogrammetry	• Wound image is taken by video camera and downloaded to a computer • Computer software calculates the length and width (area) of the wound • Software allows color images to be stored and/or printed • Noninvasive and research shows high reliability—considered the most accurate of two-dimensional measurement techniques
Wound photography	• Conventional (regular or digital) or Polaroid cameras can be used • Quality of the image varies and color of image may be distorted—depending on equipment and technique employed • Images show size of wound, color of tissue, status of surrounding skin • Images must be taken from same distance each time and ideally the same position • A suitable camera and a nurse skilled in its use is essential or images will not be reliable • Refer to discussion of wound photography and risk management below
Wound tracings	• Transparent paper is used to trace the perimeter of the wound • Reliability is affected by consistency of method used • May be effected by position of resident • Nurses may have difficulty finding and tracing the wound edge • Provides a rough estimate of the size of the external wound opening and, when serial tracings are done, shows changes in wound shape
Linear measurements	• Paper or plastic ruler used to measure length x width of wound • Irregularly shaped wound may result in nurses measuring different areas of the wound—making comparison difficult • Two-dimensional linear measurement does not acknowledge wound depth

Two-dimensional measurement techniques (see Figure 5.6 on previous page) include wound tracings, wound photography, stereophotogrammetry, linear measurements, and planimetry.

Wound photography and risk management

Recommendations vary greatly regarding wound photography as it relates to risk management. This topic should be discussed with your hospital's legal advisor and risk manager.

Some experts discourage wound photography because variation, in technique, equipment, and skill of nurses performing it often creates a risk-management problem. These problems are further compounded by the lack of adequate lighting often encountered at the bedside.

Photos that are not good clinical representations of the wound pose unnecessary challenges when mounting a legal defense. Even with digital images, the same issues of technique, training, and retention of photos arise. Additionally, digital images can easily be manipulated, which, although legally and clinically inappropriate, creates additional risk.

Three-dimensional measurement techniques

Three-dimensional techniques include linear measurements, wound molds, and fluid instillation (see Figure 5.7). The three-dimensional measurement technique includes assessing the length, width, and depth of the wound (two-dimensional techniques do not assess depth). Wounds with depth, particularly Stage III or Stage IV wounds, require such assessment.

Wound measurement: Three-dimensional linear

At minimum, measure pressure ulcers on initial admission/readmission and on a weekly basis. If the wound deteriorates, reevaluate the treatment plan as soon as the deterioration is noted. Measure the length, width, and depth of the wound, and record them in centimeters. In documentation, record length first, followed by width and depth. For example, 3.2 cm x 2.1 cm x 0.8 cm means the length of the wound is 3.2 cm, the width of the wound is 2.1 cm, and the depth of the wound is 0.8 cm.

Measure length and width of the wound in the following ways:
- Measure **distance** from wound edge to wound edge using a linear wound-measurement tool.
  - Avoid using tools that have concentric circles that would be placed over wounds. It is very difficult to visualize the wound edges with these tools, which makes accurate

FIGURE 5.7	**Three-Dimensional Measurement Techniques**

Wound molds	• A substance is placed in wound and when thickened is removed and placed in a liquid beaker (like a dental mold)
	• The amount of fluid displaced is assessed
	• Mold must be stored in specific way to avoid drying out and prevent bacterial growth
	• Time consuming process not amenable to extended care
Fluid instillation	• Instill a measured amount of saline into the wound and fill it to the wound edge; extract the fluid by syringe and measure the amount
	• Can be difficult to do depending on the location of the wound on the body
	• When done over a period of time you can assess changes in the size (volume) of the wound cavity
Linear measurement	• Measures length, width, and depth
	• May be less reliable with irregularly shaped wounds
	• Most commonly used wound measurement method in extended care (see discussion below)

measurement difficult.

- **Length** is measured using a head-to-toe reference and should be measured at the area of greatest length. A mental or written reference to clock positions may be helpful (i.e., 12:00 is the head; 6:00 is the feet). (*Note:* More than one length measurement may be obtained for irregularly shaped wounds, but documentation must reflect what was measured. Sometimes a hand drawing or tracing can be helpful with such wounds.)

- **Width** is measured in the direction of hip-to-hip and should be measured at the area of greatest width. (Refer to previous note for irregular wound width.)

- **Depth** is measured from the wound opening straight down to the deepest point in the wound bed. If depth varies, measure different areas of the wound bed to confirm the deepest site.

    - Insert cotton-tipped applicator, preferably moistened, into the deepest portion of the wound
    - Grasp the applicator with thumb and forefinger at the point that corresponds with the skin

surface/wound margin

- Withdraw the applicator while maintaining the position of your thumb and forefinger

- Measure from the tip of the applicator to that position against a linear wound ruler

- Record the depth in centimeters

- Determine the **direction** of sinus tracts/tunneling or undermining

  - Insert a cotton-tipped applicator into the wound and gently probe to identify areas of undermining or sinus tracts

  - View the direction of the applicator as if it were a hand of the clock (12:00 aligns with the head; 6:00 aligns with the feet)

  - Move clockwise, gently probing the wound to identify any areas of undermining and tunneling and note the location

- Measure the **extent** of undermining

  - Insert a cotton-tipped applicator into the area of undermining, holding it parallel to the wound

  - Advance the applicator until you feel resistance and grasp the applicator with the thumb and forefinger at the point that corresponds with the skin surface

  - Withdraw the applicator while maintaining the position of your thumb and forefinger

  - Measure from the tip of the applicator to that position

  - Record the amount of undermining in centimeters and the location range based on the clock (i.e., 1.5 cm undermining from 2:00 to 4:00)

    - Undermining always occurs with a portion of a wound edge necessitating documentation of the area affected

    - Undermining may occur in varying degrees around the wound (note these variations)

(*Note*: An alternative method to advance the applicator until you feel resistance and then gently lift the applicator beneath the skin so the tip of the applicator is visible externally. Mark that spot, measure externally from wound edge to that spot, and document as above.)

- Measure sinus **tracts/tunnels**. A wound may have more than one tunnel, and each tunnel should be measured and documented with the exact location of the tunnel, as compared to the hands of the clock (i.e., 4 cm tunnel at 3:00, 4.6 cm tunnel at 6:00)

  - Insert the cotton-tipped applicator (moistened) into the sinus tract carefully to avoid accidental trauma to adjacent structures

  - Grasp the applicator, with thumb and forefinger, where it meets the wound edge

  - Remove the applicator keeping your thumb and forefinger in place

Pain, Nutrition, and Infection Assessment

Pain management

Pain management is important for both prevention and healing of pressure ulcers. One reason is that effective pain management may improve the patient's mobility, a key factor in pressure ulcer prevention.

There is an erroneous belief that deep pressure ulcers are not painful. Debilitated patients—particularly the elderly—with pressure ulcers may be unable to convey their pain. The Agency for Healthcare Research and Quality Acute Pain Management Guideline states, "The single most reliable indicator of the existence and intensity of acute pain—and any resultant affective discomfort or distress—is the patient's self-report."[1] Nurses must meet the challenge of assessing pain effectively in vulnerable, and sometimes nonverbal, patients.

Standard of care

According to the Joint Commission on Accreditation of Healthcare Organizations (JCAHO), hospitals have the responsibility to "recognize the rights of patients to appropriate assessment and management of pain." Thus, the JCAHO has developed specific guidelines to address the overwhelming effect that unrelieved pain has on patients, and they have the support of the American Pain Society. Although the JCAHO gives individual institutions some freedom with patient pain management (e.g., the option of which pain scale to use), the requirements are very specific.

Types of pain

In 1995, Krasner[2] proposed the Chronic Wound Pain Experience model. This model categorizes pain into three categories: noncyclic acute wound pain, cyclic acute wound pain, and chronic wound pain (see Figure 6.1).

FIGURE 6.1	**Chronic Wound Pain Experience Model**

Noncyclic acute wound pain	• Single episode acute wound pain • Example: pain of sharp debridement • Potential intervention: local or topical anesthetics before debridement
Cyclic acute wound pain	• Periodic acute wound pain that occurs as a result of treatment or interventions • Examples: daily dressing changes, repositioning • Potential interventions: pressure relief surfaces or devices, dressings that reduce pain, "time-outs" during dressing changes
Chronic wound pain	• Persistent pain that occurs without manipulation • Examples: stinging, burning, or throbbing of a wound that is not being touched • Potential interventions: scheduled analgesia, relaxation strategies, referral to chronic pain clinic

Different types of pain may require different treatments. The "one size fits all" approach is woefully inadequate. For example, the vast majority of pain intervention that occurs is simply premedicating the patient 45 minutes prior to a dressing change, and although this approach may be ideal for cyclic acute wound pain, it is suboptimal for other types. A combination of interventions may be needed to eliminate or control pain.

Cyclic acute wound pain

Another potential intervention for cyclic acute wound pain during dressing changes is a "time-out" period. This easy-to-accommodate intervention allows the patient to have a break—an opportunity to regroup—during the dressing change. A good analogy for nurses who have experienced or witnessed childbirth is the time when contractions are coming fast and furious. When a contraction ends, you quickly relax, breathe, and count your blessings for the contraction-free moment. Although you know there will be another one, the break gives you an opportunity to gather your internal resources. A brief time-out during a painful dressing change provides the patient with that essential break.

The value of a gentle approach to dressing changes and wound care cannot be overstated. Explain the procedure to the patient, carefully reposition him or her, and remove dressings with care—your actions will affect the patient's pain experience. Nurses often lift the edge of the dressing and then pull the dressing off by holding that edge, but removing a dressing in this manner creates tissue damage and causes unnecessary pain. Instead, always support the tissue when removing a dressing. Move the tissue away from the dressing rather than pulling the dressing from the tissue. Also, note that if your patients experience pain, they will be less willing to comply with dressing changes or other interventions.

Unrelieved pain ultimately may lead to limitations in movement and a decline in functional status—two factors often noted in pressure ulcer development. Also, when a patient is in pain, vasoconstriction occurs, which limits the circulation to the wound and ultimately slows healing. Although you may not be able to eliminate all wound-related pain, you can always comfort patients, show empathy, and be kind and gentle.

Chronic pain

When caring for elderly patients, keep in mind that they typically have at least one painful, chronic medical condition. Pain is often increased by immobility, improper moving, friction, and shearing. In fact, 60%–80% of patients with chronic wounds experience some pain, and 50% of patients with pressure ulcers experience pain, especially those with Stages III and IV pressure ulcers.[3]

Also note that patients with paralysis and spinal cord injury may experience persistent pain in areas that otherwise have no sensation. For example, open areas on the skin can be excruciatingly painful.

Ineffective pain management results in delayed healing, lack of compliance, and prolonged care. As a matter of course, pain subsides with healing in acute wounds, but the protracted inflammatory response seen in chronic wounds may cause an increased sensitivity in the wound (primary hyperalgesia) and the surrounding skin (secondary hyperalgesia). Additional pain during debridement, dressing changes, movement, etc., may trigger allodynia, a condition in which ordinarily nonpainful stimuli cause pain.

Also, because wounds damage nerves, over time, some patients may develop neuropathic pain, a condition in which the pain response is exaggerated. Minor sensations, such as air on a wound, light touch, or change in temperature, will evoke intense pain.

Remember that inadequate wound management contributes to wound pain as well. Such complications as infection and ischemia may also contribute to the patient's pain response.

The European Wound Management Association (EWMA) published a position statement in 2002 with recommendations for managing pain during the dressing change.[4] Consider premedicating the patient and using the newer (i.e., more advanced) dressings to decrease frequency of dressing changes. Avoid assuming that wound size affects pain, as that assumption is not accurate. A small wound can be very painful, whereas a large wound in a different patient may be described as only mildly uncomfortable. Indeed, there is no proven relationship between the intensity of pain and the type or size of the wound—pain is highly variable and individualized.[5] The results of one study revealed that the degree of pain is related to the stage of the pressure ulcer, which dispels the belief that Stage IV pressure ulcers are painless.[6]

Wound pain management

The key to managing wound pain is to regularly assess for pain those patients with open wounds and pressure ulcers using a validated pain scale. If the pain is frequent or constant, consider giving a scheduled pain medication. If the patient has an order for "as needed or as required" analgesics, give them at the earliest sign of pain; do not wait for the pain to get out of control. Remember to evaluate the patient's response to pain-relieving medication.

For optimal pain relief during dressing change, consider using the following strategies:

- Offer analgesics when pain is anticipated. Premedicate the patient at least one hour before dressing change or debridement. Evaluate the patient's response by assessing the effectiveness of the medication during the procedure. If the procedure is exceedingly painful, a stronger premedication may be needed. Another option is to use a topical product, such as one containing lidocaine. Such products are highly effective but take approximately two hours to work.

- Dispel myths and teach the patient facts about pain and pain management. For example, the old adage, "no pain, no gain," is a myth. Teach the patient that in wound healing, less pain means more gain. Another common myth is that responsiveness to pain decreases with age. Many nurses believe that pain tolerance decreases, and elderly patients increase their complaints. But sensory processing of painful stimuli does not change with age. Older adults experience many painful chronic diseases. Indeed, they may experience more pain than younger adults.

- Involve the patient in decision-making, and give him or her a sense of personal control over the pain.

- Provide antianxiety medications, if requested by the patient.

- During the dressing change, monitor the patient's body language and nonverbal cues carefully for signs of pain.

- Avoid unnecessary manipulation of the wound. Protect it from sources of irritation, including air flow from a fan or window.

- Warm the cleansing solution prior to cleansing the wound, if possible.

- Use only normal saline or pH-neutral wound cleansers. Be gentle when cleaning the wound.

- Allow the patient to stop and rest during a painful procedure, such as a dressing change. Agree on a signal in advance.

- Match the dressing and treatment product to the wound. Use dressings that are nonadherent and reduce pain. Avoid woven cotton gauze, which is highly irritating to sensitive skin.

- Select wound products that maintain a moist environment in the wound bed. Do not allow the wound to become desiccated.

- Select treatments that can remain in place for a prolonged period of time. Avoid frequent dressing changes by using advanced products, if possible.

- Consider contact-layer dressings that remain in place. Doing so decreases the need to manipulate the tender wound bed and cause increased pain.

- Use compression bandages, if needed, to reduce edema and relieve pain.

- Apply barrier products to protect the wound margins, thus preventing maceration and further breakdown. This is particularly important if chemical debriding agents are being used.

- Allow the patient to remove his or her own dressing, if desired.

- Remove tape and dressings carefully and gently. If the dressing or tape sticks to the skin during dressing removal, apply normal saline, then wait a few minutes.

- Minimize the use of tape if the patient's skin is sensitive, or if he or she is at risk for skin tears. Instead, use bandage, Montgomery straps, Coban, etc., to cover the dressings.

- Follow manufacturers' instructions for removal of hydrocolloids and transparent films.

- Splint or immobilize the wound during movement and treatment, if possible.

- Teach patients to use relaxation and distraction techniques, such as guided imagery, slow, deep breathing, biofeedback, and listening to comforting music through a headset.

Pain management tip

Provide pain management by eliminating mechanical sources of pain (e.g., choosing a dressing that can be changed once daily v. multiple changes during the day; adjusting the support surface/repositioning plan). Collaborate with the patient's physician regarding analgesia and, if pain is severe, talk to the physician about a pain management service consultation, if available. Remember: New onset pain may be a sign of wound infection.

Nutritional assessments

Malnutrition and pressure ulcers often coexist in patients, but research has not determined a definite causal relationship. That is, it has shown that pressure ulcers are more frequently found in malnourished patients, but not all malnourished patients develop ulcers.

Nutritional evaluation is not a one-time event. Elderly patients, in particular, often have fluctuating nutritional status, which necessitates ongoing evaluation. Reassessment of your patient's status is essential to confirming the effectiveness of the nutritional plan of care, especially when wound healing is required.

Protein intake

Bergstrom and Braden,[7] for example, report that in their study, patients with pressure ulcers consumed 93% of the recommended daily intake of protein, whereas patients without pressure ulcers consumed 119% of the recommended daily protein. These data suggest that low dietary protein intake may predict pressure ulcer development. Although the relationship is not necessarily causal, the two are at least associated.

Protein status

Another key concept in nutritional assessment is protein status and how it relates to nitrogen balance and wound healing. With normal nutritional status, there is a balance—known as nitrogen balance—between the body's intake and loss of protein. Protein is essential to wound healing, so a negative nitrogen balance results in tissue breakdown (i.e., catabolism). Building tissue (i.e., anabolism) and repairing pressure ulcers requires a positive nitrogen balance.

Draining pressure ulcers lose protein, often at a time when protein is needed most. Even a sufficient or normal dietary intake of protein may not be enough to keep the patient in the positive nitrogen balance needed.

A person requires approximately 0.8 grams of protein per kilogram per 24 hours. In the presence of a wound, the protein requirement increases to approximately 1.25–1.5 grams per kilogram per 24 hours and approximately 35–40 kilocalories per kg of body weight per day. Thus, all patients with wounds need a thorough nutritional assessment that includes a review of the patient's history, physical examination, and laboratory work.

Serum protein levels

One aspect of nutritional assessment is assessing serum protein levels. Typically, ordering blood work for albumin or prealbumin levels assesses these levels (transferrin is another available measure of protein status, but it is ordered less frequently). Due to its lower cost, serum albumin seems to be the preferred test of medical staff, but prealbumin is a better indicator of the current status of your patient (and new technology has made the cost difference minimal).

Both tests assess visceral protein status, but there is an important difference in their half-lives—the time it takes for a measurable 50% decrease—that should be considered in the context of the patient. Albumin has a long half-life—18–21 days—and does not reflect rapid changes in nutritional status. If the patient has had a recent acute event affecting nutrition, for example, the albumin level may not detect the effects of that change. Prealbumin has a short half-life—two days—and it responds quickly to any decline in the intake of protein or calories. Thus, prealbumin is an excellent indicator of recent nutritional changes.

The following examples may help you understand the clinical application of this information.

> **Case #1**
>
> **Mrs. Shaw has had a poor appetite for several months and has experienced gradual and consistent weight loss. She was admitted to the hospital today with sudden onset of shortness of breath. During your admission assessment, you discover that she has a sacral pressure ulcer. A comprehensive nutritional assessment is being conducted. Which test is appropriate?**
>
> *Answer*: Either albumin or prealbumin would accurately detect nutritional status. Because there has not been an "acute" change and nutritional decline has occurred over a longer period of time, serum albumin levels likely would be ordered.
>
> **Case #2**
>
> **Mr. Smith was in good general health, living at home with his wife, and enjoyed an active lifestyle. He suffered a debilitating stroke and was hospitalized for five days prior to being admitted to your rehabilitation unit. Upon admission, you note that he has a pressure ulcer on his right heel. A nutrition assessment is conducted. Which test is most appropriate?**
>
> Answer: Prealbumin is the most appropriate test for this patient. Because it has a short half-life, it will show the effect of the acute health changes in this previously robust man. In this scenario, an albumin level would show you his nutritional status from when he was at home, healthy, and leading an active life.

Figure 6.2 depicts important characteristics, normal ranges, and abnormal values of blood tests that may be conducted to assess visceral protein status.

Hydration status

A patient's hydration status can affect the validity of test results for albumin and prealbumin. Dehydration will produce falsely elevated serum levels, which means that a patient with protein malnutrition may falsely show normal values. On the other hand, overhydration will produce false negative values, resulting in a patient with adequate protein showing abnormal values.

Obese patients

Nutritional assessment is equally important in obese patients. Nurses are often surprised when queried about the nutrition of a significantly overweight patient—malnutrition in such a patient often goes uninvestigated. Calorie needs for wound repair are directly related to weight and need to be incorporated into nutritional-care planning. Obese patients are at risk for delayed healing and infection because fat

FIGURE 6.2	Blood Test Characteristics to Assess Visceral Protein Status		
	Serum Albumin	**Pre-Albumin**	**Serum Transferrin**
Half-life	20 days	48 hours	7 days
"Normal ranges"	3.5–5 g/dl	15–25 mg/dl	>200 mg/dl
Moderate depletion	2.8–3.5	11–14	160–200
Severe depletion	<2.8	<11	<160

tissue is not as well perfused as muscle tissue. Additionally, many medical problems that may affect wound healing often accompany obesity.

Assessment for infection

Infection is one common chronic pressure ulcer complication, but it is difficult to assess and confirm, because most wound cultures can take 24–48 hours to provide preliminary results. This often leads to empirical treatment of presumed, but not confirmed, infections—essentially saying, "If it walks like a duck and looks like a duck, it's a duck," even when it's not. Thus, empirical treatment is not optimal, due to difficulty of assessment.

Pressure ulcers have three possible microbiologic states: *contamination*, *colonization*, and *infection*. **Contamination** is the presence in the wound of organisms that are not able to multiply in there. All chronic wounds are contaminated, and wound healing still occurs in the wound. **Colonization** is the presence of replicating (i.e., multiplying) microorganisms that adhere to the wound but are not causing injury to the host (i.e., your patient). Colonization is common, and most of the organisms are normal skin flora like *Staphylococcus epidermis*. **Infection**, however, is the presence within the pressure ulcer of replicating microorganisms that cause injury to the patient—that is, the presence and type of microorganisms overwhelm the patient's capacity to resist. Typical infectious organisms include *Staphylococcus aureus*, Beta-hemolytic *Streptococcus*, *E. coli*, *Proteus*, *Klebsiella*, *Anaerobes*, and *Pseudomonas*.

The age of the wound often corresponds to the type of microorganisms noted. In a new wound, normal skin flora is predominant, although *Staphylococcus aureus* and Beta-hemolytic strept come shortly thereafter. About a month after wound onset, anaerobic gram-negative rods—often *Proteus*, *E. coli*, and *Klebsiella*—set up housekeeping (i.e., colonize) in the wound.

The move from colonization to infection occurs as a result of the number of organisms, their virulence, and the patient's resistance to infection. Certain patient-specific systemic factors affect resistance and increase chances of wound infection. Some of these factors include edema, malnutrition, diabetes, corticosteroids, and vascular disease. Therefore, it is easy to see why elderly patients are at high risk of infection.

How do you know when a wound is infected? The most common denominators are the failure of the wound to heal and progressive deterioration of the wound. Signs and symptoms of localized infection include erythema, edema, peri-wound heat, purulent drainage, foul odor, and an increase of pain in the wound. You also may observe changes in the appearance of granulation tissue. It may appear discolored and become friable and highly prone to bleeding. In addition to these changes, localized systemic signs of infection include elevated white blood cell count and elevated body temperatures. You also may observe general malaise, mental confusion, or loss of appetite in the patient.

Not all signs and symptoms must be present to suspect infection; in fact, many elderly patients do not run temperatures even when wound sepsis has occurred. Often, frail elderly do not have an ability to mount an adequate inflammatory response.

The gold standard for diagnosing wound infection is using quantitative cultures of living wound tissue or wound fluid through needle biopsy.[7] The key to culturing is obtaining **tissue** or **tissue fluid**, not just the surface fluid or exudate. In some hospitals, however, you are often dependent on swab cultures, which typically only examine surface fluid and exudates.

When using a swab culture, thoroughly cleanse the wound before obtaining the culture. It is generally recommended that a sterile calcium alginate swab or rayon swab be used. Although it may be tempting to roll the swab in a pool of exudate and send it on its way, doing so is counterproductive. The microorganisms in that collection are usually already dead, as pus is a collection of white blood cells that have done their work and died. Therefore, after cleaning the wound, fluid can be gently expressed by pressing the swab on clean granulation tissue.

Another method commonly used is the multipoint surface swab culture. After cleaning the wound, wipe the swab across various points to detect microorganisms that may inhabit different parts. As you can probably deduce, this method primarily detects surface contaminants. Instead, by obtaining quantitative bacterial cultures of the soft tissue, you can determine whether the presence of bacteria is high enough to impair healing.

Not all infected pressure ulcers require systemic antibiotics. Localized infections, for example, generally respond to topical antibiotics. Ideally, the topical antibiotic should be effective against gram-negative, gram-positive, and anaerobic organisms. Triple antibiotic and silver sulfadiazine are good choices.[8] Always consult with the physician, document the presenting signs and symptoms, and record the wound and patient response to treatment.

Systemic antibiotics are needed, however, for systemic infections such as bacteremia, sepsis, cellulites and osteomyelitis. This complication is reported in up to 38% of patients with infected pressure ulcers. Although x-rays are typically used to diagnose osteomyelitis, plain x-rays do not reliably differentiate true osteomyelitis from pressure changes to the bone. In addition, computed tomography is more reliable than radionucleide studies, which have a high false-positive rate. No test, however, is as effective as needle biopsy of the bone. Aggressive testing for osteomyelitis is not frequently conducted, so be aware that a negative x-ray does not conclusively rule out osteomyelitis.

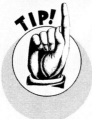

Infection control tip

Avoid exogenous sources of contamination, such as urinary/fecal incontinence. Exposure to feces will increase the level of bacterial colonization in a pressure ulcer.

Remember: The assessment is the basis for subsequent treatment, documentation, and evaluation, and it is critical for your assessment to go beyond wound measurements. Your assessment as a whole gives life to the wound description, which prevents you from shortchanging your patients or underutilizing your clinical skills. Risk management in this context involves assessing and managing both the patient and your professional risk.

References

1. Acute Pain Management Guideline Panel. 1992. Acute pain management: Operative or medical procedures and trauma. Clinical Practice Guideline #1. Rockville, MD: Public Health Service, U.S. Department of Health and Human Services. p. 11.

2. Krasner, D. 1995. The chronic wound pain experience: a conceptual model. *Ostomy Wound Management* 41(3): 20.

3. European Wound Management Society. 2002. Position document: Pain at wound dressing changes. London, UK: Medical Education Partnership Ltd., 2, 8.

4. Szor J.K., and C. Bourguignon. 1999. Description of pressure ulcer pain at rest and at dressing change. *Journal of Wound Ostomy, and Continence Nursing* 26: 115–20.

5. Coleman, K. 2001. Practical management of skin tears. *Woundcare Network* Issue 6.

6. Bergstrom, N., and B. Braden. 1992. A prospective study of pressure sore risk among institutionalized elderly. *Journal of the American Geriatric Society* 40: 747–758.

7. Perry C., R. Pearson, and G. Miller. 1991. Accuracy of cultures of material from swabbing of the superficial aspect of the wound and needle biopsy in the preoperative assessment of osteomyelitis. *Journal of Bone and Joint Surgery (American)* 73(5): 745–749.

8. National Pressure Ulcer Advisory Panel. Frequently asked questions: wound infection and infection control. *www.npuap.org* (accessed on July 2000).

Treatment Concepts

Before developing a treatment plan for pressure ulcers, understand some basic concepts. Treatment does not refer only to a topical approach to the wound; it involves the total interdisciplinary approach. Where do you start?

First, define the overall goal of treatment. Interdisciplinary teams sometimes get lost in this process—they meet and each team member discusses his or her specialized area separately. Such care plans become routine and are problem- or disease-based instead of patient-based. When that happens, you have missed the point of a total interdisciplinary approach.

There is a tremendous amount of literature and seminars that cover pressure ulcer management and treatment, but the overall goal of treatment is rarely emphasized or even discussed. This omission likely stems from a tendency to focus thought processes on the wound itself.

Instead, treatment must occur within the context of the patient's whole situation. Determine whether the goal is healing, maintenance, or comfort. Then, armed with this information, your team can develop a plan that is consistent with the goal.

Treatment goals

The overall goals of treatment are to promote wound healing, prevent complications, prevent deterioration of the existing wound, prevent additional skin breakdown, and minimize the harmful effects of the wound on the patient's overall condition. For any given situation, however, you also must evaluate the parameters within which you are working: Are there advance directives that limit the scope or selection of wound treatments? Is it likely that the wound will heal? Have you discussed with the patient and the interdisciplinary team the risks and benefits of treatments you are considering? Ultimately, the treatment plan will depend on your patient's wishes, condition, and prognosis, in addition to the reversibility of the wound.

Divide goals into three main categories: *comfort, maintenance,* and *healing.* If the primary goal is comfort, it doesn't make sense to initiate an aggressive wound-healing program for a patient who is experiencing pain that can't be well-managed during dressing changes. The interdisciplinary team, the patient, and the patient's family must determine the goals of care.

How do you determine this goal of care? Generally, you know when healing is realistic: when there is no terminal diagnosis and the patient's underlying physical condition is one that you likely can rehabilitate or stabilize. Maintenance may be the appropriate goal for a patient with a chronic wound, an irreversible underlying medical condition, or a gradual decline in health status and function. Such a patient is not considered terminal but, due to his or her gradual decline, may have difficulty healing to the point of complete closure. For a patient with a terminal condition, a comfort goal is the most appropriate choice. This patient may be losing weight despite your best efforts, body systems may be shutting down, and the patient's condition is expected to worsen.

Whichever goal you choose will guide you in treatment decisions. If comfort is the priority, place your emphasis on quality-of-life issues. Pain management is important, and choosing treatments that are comforting and do not require frequent changing are good choices. Also, remember to manage wound odor, which is another important quality-of-life concern.

Treatment plan

Once you have agreed on a goal, you are ready to start a *treatment plan.* Make a conscious decision to think in these terms. Wound management is not just the treatment product you apply: It must be a comprehensive approach based on the expertise of the interdisciplinary team members and accepted standards of practice. It should include

- ✔ repositioning schedule in chair and in bed, as well as back-to-bed routines
- ✔ positioning devices, including contracture management
- ✔ pressure-relief devices for chair/bed
- ✔ interventions to reduce friction and shear—including but not limited to moisturizing skin, protecting heels, drawing sheets for lifting, limiting head-of-bed elevation (if possible), etc.
- ✔ management of incontinence, including, if possible, bowel/bladder program/incontinence skin barriers and briefs/underpads

✔ medical assessment and treatment of complicating or contributing history or diagnoses
✔ nutrition, including consideration of labs, vitamin support, and protein supplementation, as indicated
✔ hydration management (if needed)
✔ pain-management needs
✔ psychosocial support
✔ education of and communication with the patient/responsible party
✔ wound-cleansing product
✔ topical treatment determined by wound and patient needs
✔ dressings that provide a moist wound environment
✔ keeping peri-wound skin dry, controlling exudates, and in the case of a cavity wound, eliminating dead space
✔ weekly reassessment of the wound, at a minimum, and revision of the treatment plan as needed

Consider taking additional steps, depending on the patient's specific needs to ensure you are doing everything possible to maximize the patient's healing potential.

Treating the wound

After initiating the interdisciplinary assessment, you are ready to start treating the wound. There are a variety of conceptual topics and categories of products to discuss.

Moist healing

For those of you who have been nurses for many years, you probably remember using heat lamps to treat pressure ulcers. At that time, the collective wisdom said that it was best to air and dry it out. For those of you who have been nurses for a *really* long time, you may remember the skin of the buttocks being taped to the raised siderails of the bed. The intent was to expose the sacral pressure area to the air and the heat lamp. Given the regulatory environment and the virtual prohibition of siderails, it is a good thing this practice was later disproved through scientific research.

In the 1960s, wound researcher George Winter determined that moist wounds heal faster than dry wounds. Numerous researchers have since confirmed this finding. Moisture improves the collagen synthesis needed for tissue repair and allows for migration of the epithelial cells. A moist wound environment also reduces pain and produces less scarring.

However, even 44 years later, nurses do not embrace moist healing consistently. Heat lamps are rarely used, but there is still a disparity between research and daily practice. For example, despite the countless moisture retentive dressings available, many hospitals continue to rely on gauze dressings due to cost or lack of understanding. Cost, of course, is a relative term—yes, gauze dressings are cheaper on a unit-purchase basis than are most moisture retentive dressings, but prolonged healing and nursing time make the cost difference less impressive.

How do you know what moisture-retentive dressings are, and how do you compare them? First, understand a moisture vapor transmission rate (MVTR). The MVTR is the degree to which dressings dry the wound. To maintain a moist wound environment, an MVTR of less than 35 grams of water vapor per square meter per hour is required. You do not need to know how to do the calculations because various dressing manufacturers study the MVTR, but you must understand the difference between good and bad MVTRs so you can make comparative selections.

For example, standard woven gauze has an MVTR of 68. If you compare that number to the desired MVTR of less than 35, it is clear why gauze is not an ideal choice. By comparison, most hydrocolloid dressings have an MVTR of 8. One word of caution: Maceration of the skin can occur if the dressing is not permeable to water vapor at all. There needs to be a balance between moist healing and water vapor permeability to prevent wound fluid from accumulating and macerating the skin. The bottom line: If the dressing material transmits more moisture vapor than the wound loses, the wound will dry out.

Wound cleansing and irrigation

The proper methods of and products for wound cleaning are somewhat controversial. Some believe wound irrigation will disrupt new tissue formation, while others believe it is essential. Some experts support thorough cleaning of the wound and irrigation at proper pressures and conclude that irrigation minimizes pressure ulcer colonization and improves healing. Regardless of how you believe is best to do it, the key is to use irrigation pressures efficiently to remove debris but not disturb healthy new granulation tissue.

The Agency for Healthcare Research and Quality (AHRQ) guidelines recommend using nontoxic cleansing agents. Topical antiseptics like sodium hypochlorite (Dakin's solution), acetic acid, and hydrogen peroxide are not recommended: When tested, these agents were found to be toxic to granulation tissue. Note that the tests were conducted with full-strength solutions, although hydrogen peroxide in any dilution is not recommended—there is concern that it may cause air emboli. Some health practitioners recommend diluted sodium hypochlorite or acetic acid to manage Pseudomonas or Staphylococcal colonization, but be careful with this practice because it is contrary to the AHRQ guidelines for the treatment of pressure ulcers.

Most wounds can be cleaned adequately using normal saline or sterile water. If you use a commercial wound cleanser, check its toxicity to granulating wound tissue. Many products were tested and reported in the AHRQ guidelines, and studies have been conducted to determine the required amount of dilution for many wound cleansers. Specifically, these studies have focused on the cleansing agents' effect on blood-cell viability and phagocytic function, and their results showed wide variation. The 1997 evaluation of 10 commercial wound cleansers showed that all had deleterious effects on the tissue and phagocytic activity unless diluted.[1] Some products needed dilution at a ratio of 1:10, while others needed dilution at a ratio of 1:1,000.

The Food and Drug Administration does not regulate wound cleansers, so be an educated consumer. Wound cleansers do have benefits over normal saline when the wound has adherent materials because the surfactants in commercial wound cleansers often help remove these materials. In general, however, normal saline is the preferred wound cleaner. It adequately cleans most wounds, is not harmful to tissue, and is physiologic.

Another factor to consider when irrigating is the temperature of the solution. Often saline bottles are stored in back rooms or closed treatment rooms with cooler temperatures. But cleansing with cool solution can cause hypothermia of the wound, which can lead to slow healing and impair the immune response. One study found that local tissue temperatures were reduced for up to 40 minutes after cleaning the wound. Mitosis and leukocyte activities were reduced for up to three hours.

Irrigation of the wound with normal saline is an effective cleansing technique with safe irrigation pressures. The recommended range for irrigation pressure is between 4 and 15 pounds per square inch (psi). Pressures below 4 psi are too low to clean the wound effectively; pressures above 15 psi will be detrimental to the wound. A psi of 8 is ideal because it cleans the wound and reduces the risk of wound trauma. A 35-ml syringe (with an angiocath to avoid risk of a needlestick) provides an 8 psi irrigation-pressure stream. Pressures at the higher recommended range may be needed in the presence of slough or eschar, but above 15 psi, they can cause wound trauma and will drive bacteria into the tissue. Prepackaged canisters of pressurized saline are a good option because they rely on saline as the wound irrigant and ensure the appropriate range of pressure.

Pulsatile lavage is a method of wound irrigation in which a machine provides intermittent delivery of irrigation solution to the wound surface. Many of these machines combine irrigation with suction to remove the irrigation solution and wound debris. Take precautions when using such machines, especially if using high pressures or applying pulse lavage to the wound of a patient on anticoagulant therapy. If bleeding occurs, discontinue the irrigation.

Physicians sometimes prescribe a whirlpool for irrigating large wounds or those with significant necrosis in a body part that can be immersed. Typically, after a whirlpool treatment, the wound is rinsed forcefully. However, research to support whirlpool use is limited, and the benefits initially attributed to the whirlpool are now questioned. The decrease in surface bacteria is now believed to be due to the post-whirlpool irrigation rather than the whirlpool itself.

Cross-contamination is another large concern with this procedure. Even when an antiseptic solution is added to the water, you must be concerned with the effects of the antiseptic on the tissue. Another concern is the position of the wound in relation to the high-pressure water jets in the whirlpool—if it is too close, the jets may cause trauma to the wound. For these reasons, the risks associated with the whirlpool often outweigh the benefits.

Debridement

Debridement is essential in almost all wounds with nonviable tissue. The main exception is stable necrotic heel ulcers. If there is dry, black eschar on the heel, it should not be debrided unless it is tender, is fluctuant, has erythema, or is draining (see photograph # 7, *Heel with eschar*, on your laminated insert). If these conditions are not present, do not debride the heel. The AHRQ guideline reports that the eschar is believed to provide a natural protective cover. If the wound starts to show signs of the above complications, however, debridement has to occur.

Heel eschar will sometimes change over time, necessitating a change in treatment approach. If you observe a stable eschar on the heel that does not show signs of complications, off-load the foot to eliminate pressure. You may opt to apply a protective dry dressing. In this case, monitor the eschar daily, and if a complication like drainage occurs, initiate an active treatment to debride the wound.

Another contraindication for debridement is stable (i.e., neither fluctuant, draining, nor infected) ischemic wounds or those with dry gangrene. Debridement is primarily contraindicated due to poor blood perfusion to the extremity where the ischemic wound is located. These wounds do not have origins in pressure and therefore will not be discussed in detail in this book.

General debridement methods

For pressure ulcers, four general debridement methods may be used alone or in combination with one another: autolytic, chemical, mechanical, and sharp debridement. These methods are differentiated by their selectivity. Nonselective debridement takes both living and dead tissue out of the wound. In selective debridement, only the dead, necrotic tissue is removed.

- Autolytic debridement: Selective
- Chemical (enzyme) debridement: Selective
- Mechanical debridement: Nonselective
- Sharp debridement: May be selective or nonselective

The method of debridement chosen is dictated by many factors, including the amount of necrotic tissue, presence or absence of infection, condition of the wound, condition of the patient, and access to or availability of services. Regardless of which type you use, debridement is an essential component of treatment for necrotic wounds. The nurse and physician must be knowledgeable about the advantages and disadvantages of each method and use the one that is most consistent with the goal of treatment and the patient's overall condition.

Sharp debridement

Properly trained nurses, certified in conservative sharp debridement, may do it if the hospital policy and the state allow it within these nurses' scope of practice. Sharp debridement is the most efficient method for removal of necrotic tissue and is the most desired option if infection is present. Because this procedure can be uncomfortable for the patient, provide analgesia. After sharp debridement, use dry dressings for eight to 24 hours to limit bleeding. Next, begin to apply moist dressings.

Mechanical debridement

Mechanical debridement typically means wet-to-dry debridement. It involves applying saline-moistened gauze to the wound bed and allowing it to dry. Once dry, the dressing is pulled off the wound. When employing this method of debridement, carefully consider the type of gauze you use. The most effective is open-weave cotton gauze; nonwoven gauze is not usually effective because its composition does not allow the tissue to adhere to it.

When removing such a dressing, do not moisten it to facilitate removal. The purpose of this method is to remove the wound debris and necrosis mechanically. Thus, moistening of the gauze is counterproductive. Many experts view mechanical debridement as the least desirable option because it is nonselective and generally painful for the patient. That is, it may remove the debris, but it is harmful to good wound tissue as well.

Although physicians often order wet-to-dry mechanical debridement, less painful and less traumatic options are available. A good analogy to that debridement method is eyebrow waxing—it may be effective in removing the hair, but would you opt to do it two or three times a day if other options were available? Discontinue use of wet-to-dry dressings when the heavy eschar is removed so that viable tissue is not continually traumatized.

Autolytic debridement

Autolytic debridement requires keeping the wound moist. It typically involves using synthetic dressings to cover the wound and may include the addition of wound gels or moisture-depositing products. Autolytic debridement allows the dead tissue to self-digest using the natural enzymes in wound fluids. It's similar to creating a crock-pot–type environment: It takes longer than other methods, but it is painless and selective. Note: This form of debridement is contraindicated if infection is present, because it provides an environment in which the microorganisms flourish.

Chemical (enzyme) debridement

Enzyme debridement involves application of a topical debriding agent to the necrotic tissue. The product penetrates the eschar and works to dissolve the necrosis. The AHRQ guidelines support cross hatching (i.e., sharp, shallow slits) of the eschar to allow full penetration of the enzyme. If you apply topical enzymes and do not see a decrease in necrotic tissue, you may want to ask the physician or nurse practitioner to crosshatch the eschar.

Commercially available enzymes are primarily papain/urea combinations and collagenase. Both products are generally helpful with debridement, but papain-urea is thought to produce more efficient results. One study conducted in 2000[2] reported a greater reduction in necrotic tissue when using papain-urea (95.4%) rather than collagenase (35.8%) over a four-week period. Topical debridement enzymes require a physician/nurse practitioner order and are obtained from the pharmacy. A note of caution: Watch what the pharmacy sends you—generic substitutions of the product ordered are not always equivalent. The use of generic substitutions is not recommended because their efficacy has not always been established.

When you apply topical enzymes, next apply a moist dressing. This helps soften the eschar to allow for better penetration of the enzyme. The frequency of dressing change depends on the amount of exudate but typically is done either once or twice a day.

Fill dead space

The process of filling dead space in a wound typically is called "packing" because the wound is often stuffed with dressing material. However, this practice is not a good, so "loosely filling dead space" is a better objective and phrase.

The purpose of loosely filling a wound is to occupy the dead space to avoid potential abscess formation and premature closing of the wound. To do so, fluff and place the material in the wound in a manner that ensures contact with the wound base and edges—including undermining and sinus tracts. When a sinus tract is present, strip gauze is usually the preferred product because its varied widths allow you to fill narrow areas. Be careful not to overpack the wound, which could increase the pressure on the base or sides and create additional wound trauma.

Change wound dressings

Like nursing, changing wound dressings is both an art and a science. The art involves organizing your time and supplies, protecting the patient's privacy, and making the dressing change as painless as possible. The science involves preventing wound contamination or cross-contamination, thereby preventing infection. Note that in recent years, surveyors have cited nurses for improper prevention of cross-contamination. To avoid contamination of the patient and the environment, practice the seven correct—or "right"—patient and procedure indicators during dressing changes.

Seven rights

The seven "rights" for dressing changes are as follows:

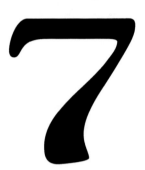

Right patient
Right amount/quantity
Right dressing
Right environment
Right time
Right technique
Right treatment product

Clean v. sterile dressings

Over the years, practice has moved away from sterile technique and sterile dressings. Because pressure ulcers are nonsterile wounds, they do not require sterile technique unless required by your hospital policy. Open wounds are contaminated with microorganisms already, so just be careful to not donate extra ones. A patient with a moist wound in which white blood cells can function effectively and who has adequate immunity is safe with clean technique. The AHRQ pressure ulcer-treatment guidelines state, "Use clean dressings, rather than sterile ones, to treat pressure ulcers, as long as dressing procedures comply with institutional infection control guidelines."[3]

To be considered "clean," clean dressings must be stored appropriately. Retain the dressing in the original packaging or other protective wrap to minimize the risk of dust accumulation or contamination—clean dressings require vigilance to ensure that contamination does not occur. Wash the treatment surface before and after the procedure. In addition, handwashing is required prior to donning clean, nonsterile gloves at all steps of the pressure ulcer care—prior to removing the dressing, after removing the dressing and changing gloves in preparation for applying the new dressing, and upon completion of the dressing change. If treating multiple pressure ulcers on the same patient, start with the cleanest wound and end with the most contaminated.

Be especially careful of potential cross-contamination between you and wound-care products. After you have touched the wound, do not come in contact with supplies or irrigant containers that are not being used specifically for that patient at that time.

The concern over cross-contamination naturally links to a brief discussion of locating treatment carts in patient rooms: Doing so may be an infection-control disaster waiting to happen. Many organizations advocate taking the treatment cart into the patient room for access to supplies and using the top of it as a treatment surface. However, many experts disagree with this practice. The likelihood of cross-contamination is so high that the benefit of its accessibility does not outweigh the risks. Indeed, when the carts are in the rooms, nurses are more apt to go back into a drawer with gloves on after forgetting a treatment item. Drawers may be left ajar, potentially contaminating products within. Compounding these problems is the lack of adequate or effective cleaning of the treatment cart surface pre- and post-treatment. For these reasons, strongly consider the advantages and disadvantages of this practice and ensure that your facility protocols include the necessary safeguards.

Removing the dressing

When removing the patient's dressing, the procedure should be as gentle—and sterile—as possible. Therefore, before removing a soiled dressing, always wash your hands and apply clean gloves. Then, hold traction on the skin with one hand while carefully loosening the edges of the tape with the other hand. Gently remove the dressing. If it sticks to the wound, pour a small amount of sterile saline on the dressing. Let it sit for a minute and then gently remove it, holding gentle traction on the skin above the wound. Note the color, odor, and amount of drainage. Discard the soiled dressing in a plastic bag placed at the foot of the bed and away from clean supplies or according to hospital policy. Use tape remover or baby oil to remove remaining adhesive from the skin.

Nutritional and vitamin support

Although there are a range of opinions on the type and dosage of recommended vitamins, there is general agreement that nutritional deficiencies must be corrected as part of your treatment plan.

Calorie and protein supplementation

In 2003, the National Pressure Ulcer Advisory Panel recommended enhanced calorie and protein supplementation for underweight patients or for those experiencing weight loss. Protein or calorie malnutrition affect fibroblast proliferation and collagen synthesis, which interfere with wound repair. Beyond the recommended 35–40 kcalories per kg of body weight per day for total calories and 1.0–1.5 g protein per kg of body weight per day for total protein, you may want to consider other support. *Note*: Some clinicians support a protein per kg range of up to 2 g of protein per kg per day.

Vitamins

Opinions and research vary on the need for, type of, and dosage of vitamins. Even the research on vitamin C and zinc, vitamins commonly ordered to promote wound healing, is confusing and conflicting. If there is not agreement on vitamin support, why is it routinely included? Because in most cases, moderate supplementation will not cause harm. The AHRQ guidelines suggest giving vitamin and mineral supplements if deficiencies are confirmed or suspected. It also references research that concludes that vitamin and mineral deficiencies have been demonstrated in the majority of patients in nursing homes.

Vitamin C

Vitamin C, for example, is associated with wound healing because it is necessary for collagen formation and it gives tensile strength to new collagen. Vitamin C is a water-soluble vitamin, which means it is not stored in the body and it needs to be replenished on a daily basis. The recommended daily allowance (RDA) for healthy adults is 75 mg for females and 90 mg for males. The AHRQ guidelines state that supplemental vitamins may be needed in levels up to 10 times the RDA when specific deficiencies are diagnosed. This means a range of 750 mg per day (for women) or 900 mg per day (for men) may be needed. The National Academy of Sciences-National Research Council (NAS-NRC) RDA indicates that the upper limit for vitamin C is 2,000 mg per day. Given AHRQ and NAS-NRC literature, it is reasonable to provide vitamin C in the range of 500–1,000 mg. This is enough to ensure an adequate supply, but it does not reach levels under which adverse effects could occur.

Zinc

Zinc supplementation is more controversial. Although zinc has a known role in collagen formation and protein synthesis, opinions vary regarding the dosage and duration of treatment—there is sufficient literature to suggest that zinc may be a double-edged sword. At recommended levels, it is believed to improve immune function, but at higher levels, it actually impairs such function. In addition, most research has shown no improvement in wound healing with zinc supplementation unless there is a zinc deficiency (which is usually not known). The Food and Drug Administration RDA of zinc is 15 mg.

In wound management, zinc is often ordered as zinc sulfate 220 mg per day indefinitely. Various studies have suggested that dosages higher than 150 mg per day for more than even one week can impair immune function. The potential toxic effects of high levels, including impaired wound healing and immune function, are ample reasons for caution. Zinc in high doses also often causes gastrointestinal (GI) problems, which may manifest as a decline in appetite. Consider zinc as a possible contributor to such GI problems if high-level supplementation has been provided for a longer duration. Be careful when developing your vitamin supplementation regimen for wound healing. Limit zinc sulfate supplementation to 220 mg for two to four weeks.

Foley catheters

Some question using foley catheters to manage urinary incontinence for patients with pressure ulcers. Using foley catheters is known to create risk for development of urinary-tract infections and therefore requires careful consideration. Standards of practice and regulations provide some guidance on this matter—in general, they agree that foley catheters are not indicated for Stage II wounds but that they may be needed for Stage III/ IV wounds on the trunk.

The AHRQ "Clinical Practice Guideline Number 2 (1996 update) on Urinary Incontinence in Adults: Acute and Chronic Management" [4] says, in part, "Indwelling catheters are recommended for selected incontinent patients who are terminally ill or for patients with pressure ulcers as a short-term treatment." It provides further guidance to make it clear Stage II pressure ulcers are generally excluded: "In situations where the severity of the incontinence and the complexity of the person's care have contributed to skin irritation or pressure ulcers (Stage III/IV), an indwelling catheter may be indicated for short-term therapy until the skin condition resolves."

The WOCN's fact sheets are reviewed for scientific accuracy, appropriateness of content, and readability and are accepted standards of practice. Thus, it is more explicit in its clinical fact sheet for indwelling catheters, which contains the following information is listed on the fact sheet:

Indications for use include

- monitoring of acutely ill patients
- management of terminally or severely ill patients
- urinary retention not manageable by other means
- management of urinary incontinence in patient with Stage III or Stage IV pressure ulcers on trunk

Contraindications:

- Management of urinary incontinence not associated with full-thickness pressure ulcers on trunk
- Urinary retention that can be otherwise managed (e.g., with clean intermittent catheterization)

This fact sheet is clear: Foley catheterization should only be considered for Stage III or IV trunk wounds. The contraindication reinforces this by saying that it is contraindicated unless there are full-thickness pressure ulcers on the trunk. Full-thickness pressure ulcers are Stage III or IV only, as Stage IIs represent partial-thickness skin loss.

Individual patient assessment should always prevail, but expert consensus says that urinary catheterization is not appropriate as part of the treatment plan for Stage II pressure ulcers unless other coexisting conditions (e.g., terminal illness, urinary retention, etc.) warrant their use. Although catheterization may be appropriate in the management of Stage III/IV pressure ulcers, always assess for less-invasive means of containing urinary incontinence, when possible.

Prevention of additional ulcers

Patients who have experienced a pressure ulcer are at increased risk for suffering another. To prevent additional ulcers from developing, consider instituting the following preventative measures:

- Thoroughly cleanse the skin at the time of soiling and at routine intervals
- Use a mild cleansing agent and avoid hot water to decrease irritation and dryness of skin
- Avoid massage over bony prominences
- Minimize skin injury due to friction and shear by practicing proper positioning and turning techniques

References

1. Hellewell, T., et al. 1997. A cytotoxicity evaluation of antimicrobial and non-antimicrobial wound cleansers. *Wounds* 9(1): 15.

2. Alvarez, O.M., A. Fenandez-Obregon, R.S. Rogers, L. Bergamo, J. Masso, and M. Black. 2000. Chemical debridement of pressure ulcers: A prospective, randomized, comparative trial of collagenase and papain/urea formulations. *Wounds* 12: 15–25.

3. Treatment of Pressure Ulcers Guideline Panel 1994. Treatment of Pressure Ulcers. Clinical Practice Guidelines, No. 15. Rockville, MD: U.S. Department of Health and Human Services. Public Health Service, Agency of Health Care Policy and Research. AHCPR publication no. 95-0652.

4. Fantl, J.A., et al. 1996. Urinary Incontinence in Adults: Acute and Chronic Management. Clinical Practice Guideline No. 2, 1996 Update. Rockville, MD: U.S. Department of Health and Human Services. Public Health Service, Agency for Health Care Policy and Research. AHCPR Publication No. 96-0682.

Wound-Care Products

When it comes to choosing dressings to treat pressure ulcers, ensure that the products

- provide a moist environment
- keep the peri-wound skin dry
- control exudate (without dehydrating the wound)
- eliminate the dead space by loosely filling open spaces
- maintain consistency with patient-specific goals

What's on the market?

More than 1,000 wound-care products are available, and new ones are constantly in development. This chapter places each product into a general category and follows with a description of eac of the categories. When you understand the indications and contraindications for each of the categories, you will be able to make treatment decisions within that category based on your facility formulary.

Gauze

Gauze is available in various forms, including dry or impregnated with other materials (water, saline, etc.). Gauze can be woven, nonwoven, or consist of a synthetic blend (see Figure 8.1).

FIGURE 8.1	**Types of Gauze**
Indications	• Non-woven gauze—cleaning, wiping, absorbing, protection • Woven gauze—packing ("loosely filling") and debridement • Dry gauze can be used for surgical wounds, for post-sharp debridement to limit bleeding, and to protect dry gangrenous wounds that cannot be debrided • Impregnated gauze—hydration or absorption • May be helpful for filling large cavities or narrow tunnels
Points to ponder/ precautions	• Dry gauze will not support a moist environment • Wet-to-dry gauze debridement is painful • Wet gauze may cause maceration of surrounding tissue
Tips	• Select type of gauze based on its intended function (see above)

Transparent film dressings

Transparent film dressings are also known as moisture vapor permeable dressings (see Figure 8.2). They promote a moist environment by trapping moisture on the wound surface. The dressings are not permeable to bacteria or fluid but are semipermeable to oxygen and water vapor. These dressings are made of thin polyurethane sheets coated on one side with hypoallergenic adhesive.

Hydrogels

Hydrogel dressings are used to maintain a moist wound environment (see Figure 8.3 on p. 84). They are available in gels and sheet gels of various sizes. Hydrogel sheet dressings are soothing and often help reduce pain. These dressings may contain up to 96% water. Amorphous hydrogels are similar to the sheets, but the polymers in town are not cross-linked, so they are not as cooling as the sheet form.

FIGURE 8.2	Transparent Film Dressings
Indications	• Superficial wounds with minimal exudates • Wounds with eschar to facilitate autolytic debridement • Use in combination with an absorbing dressing, as a secondary dressing
Points to ponder/ precautions	• Used alone they have no capacity to absorb exudates • Can be damaging to fragile tissue upon removal, (i.e., causes skin stripping)
Tips	• May help on the heels of patients to minimize negative affects of friction (if you can prevent rolling) • Use skin sealant prior to apply to minimize pain and skin stripping on removal • Film dressings used for IV sites are not the same as film dressings for wounds; IV films have a higher MVTR than appropriate for wounds—do not interchange • Change dressing if exudate goes beyond the edge of the wound and you can see it on the peri-wound skin • At removal, stretch the film parallel to the wound to break the seal—do not pull upwards

FIGURE 8.3	Hydrogel Dressings
Indications	• Full-thickness wounds (Stage IIIs and IVs) primarily • Dry or minimally draining wounds • To promote autolytic debridement (when covered by film) • Painful wounds
Points to ponder/ precautions	• Not for use with moderate to heavy draining wounds • Close monitoring of the wound is needed to observe for maceration of surrounding skin or over-hydration of wound • Amorphous hydrogels become thinner at room temperature and may strike through the dressing • Some have occlusive backings and should not be used with infected wounds
Tips	• Cut the sheet forms to the size of the wound to prevent overlap onto healthy, intact skin • In deep wounds apply gel to wound base and walls with gauze to fill the space—do not just fill the depth with gel • Make your own hydrogel impregnated gauze by applying amorphous hydrogel directly to the gauze and working it through

Alginates

Alginates are primary dressings (i.e., in direct contact with the wound) and require a secondary cover dressing (see Figure 8.4). Alginates are derived from brown seaweed and are available in rope form or nonwoven pads. Calcium alginate exchanges calcium ions for sodium ions when in contact with anything containing sodium—in this case, wound exudate.

FIGURE 8.4	**Alginate Dressings**
Indications	• Wounds with moderate to heavy exudate • Wounds with visible depth needing filling • Bleeding wounds (helps achieve hemostasis)
Points to ponder/ precautions	• Not for use with low exudating wounds • Risk of drying out wound bed • Have tan mucous-like appearance when removed that is often mistaken for an infectious process
Tips	• Try different types of alginates—some have better wet strength than others and can be removed in one piece • When filling deep sinus tracts, strip packing gauze is better because it is more easily retrieved • Do not moisten before applying or you will interfere with its absorptive ability

These dressings conform to the wound size, and different types react differently at that point. Some keep their structure and are lifted out of the wound during dressing changes, while other brands become gel-like and must be irrigated from the wound. They absorb many times their own weight, but they are lightweight, so don't overestimate their capacity to absorb. Absorptive secondary dressings typically are needed for heavily exudating wounds.

Collagen dressings

Collagen dressings promote the deposit of collagen in the wound bed and come in gels, pads, and particles (see Figure 8.5). Typically, the gel forms come loaded in syringes for application in the wound. Use them in wound cavities to fill dead space and to absorb the exudates and maintain a moist environment. Use a secondary dressing with these products.

FIGURE 8.5	Collagen Dressings
Indications	• All stages of wounds (but not usually necrotic wounds) • Recalcitrant wounds
Points to ponder/ precautions	• Not indicated in dry or necrotic wounds • Formulated with Type 1 bovine collagen that is purified—cannot be used with patient sensitive to bovine products
Tips	• In minimally draining wound, use gel applied 1/4 inch thick • If wound is deep, apply gel and fill cavity with saline gauze or other primary dressing • If pad is used allow for expansion as exudate is absorbed— leave 1/4–1/2 in between the sides of the wound and the pad

Composite dressings

Composite dressings combine many properties into one dressing (see Figure 8.6). They must contain an absorbent layer, a bacterial barrier, an adhesive border, and include a nonadherent or semiadherent surface in contact with the wound. They resemble fabric-covered Band-Aids.

Contact layer dressings

A contact layer dressing is made of a polymer net that does not stick to the wound. This unique product does not need to be removed with every dressing change. The perforated or woven polymer allows wound exudate to pass through the mesh or perforations on to the secondary dressing. Change the contact layer only once a week and the secondary dressing as needed during that period (see Figure 8.7 on p. 88).

FIGURE 8.6	**Composite Dressings**
Indications	• As a primary or secondary dressing for wounds of all stages • In deep wounds a primary filler-type material is needed • Lightly draining wounds
Points to ponder/ precautions	• Not for use with heavily draining wounds
Tips	• Dressing needs to extend at least 1 in beyond all wound edges and be adhered to intact skin • Cannot be cut to size without affecting the properties of the dressing • Use skin sealant prior to applying to minimize stripping of the skin from the adhesive border during dressing removal

Foam dressings

Foam dressings are water-proof, bacteria-proof dressings made of polyurethane foam (see Figure 8.8). Some types are semiocclusive and can only be used as cover dressings; others are used to fill a wound cavity. They may be ordered with or without an adhesive border. Foam dressings were developed to improve the limited absorbency of the first film dressings. The polyurethane foam contains tiny open cells that wick wound fluid away from the wound bed and hold it.

Hydrocolloids

Hydrocolloids are typically occlusive and adhesive wafer dressings (see Figure 8.9 on p. 89). Most hydrocolloid dressings react with exudates to form a gel-type covering that maintains a moist wound environment. The size, thickness, and absorptive capability vary depending on the manufacturer. Some dressings are constructed in the shape of body contours to improve conformability and wear time. Others have tapered or "step-down" adhesive borders to decrease the incidence of rolling of the dressing edges. Some types of hydrocolloids have alginate incorporated into the dressing to enhance exudate absorption. These dressings can be used with filling pastes or powders but typically are not used for deep wounds.

FIGURE 8.7	**Contact Layer Dressings**
Indications	• Primary dressings for clean wounds
Points to ponder/ precautions	• Not recommended for dry wounds or those with thick exudates • Not for use with undermining wounds or those with sinus tracts
Tips	• The layer is placed over the wound surface like a liner • It can overlap the surrounding skin without causing damage

FIGURE 8.8	**Foam Dressings**
Indications	• For moderate to heavily draining wounds • May be used for protection of intact skin • May be used under compression dressings
Points to ponder/ precautions	• Not intended for use with dry or ischemic wounds • If used with shallow wound with minimal exudates, it may dry out the wound bed
Tips	• Some types are not as conformable and may need creativity in placement to contour certain body parts (e.g., gluteal folds) • Extend dressing at least 1 in onto intact skin • The cavity form of foam dressing is preshaped and must fit wound size and shape

FIGURE 8.9	**Hydrocolloid Dressings**
Indications	• Best for minimally draining wounds • May be used for autolytic debridement • Protection of intact skin
Points to ponder/ precautions	• Create a hypoxic wound—nonpermeable to water vapor or oxygen • Not for use with infected wounds due to occlusive properties • Not appropriate for deep wounds with or without sinus tracts • Not for use with moderate/heavy draining wounds due to limited absorptive capacity unless using type with alginate incorporated into the dressing • Maceration of peri-wound skin may occur if drainage is not contained • May "melt down" into wound and have odor—not necessarily indicative of infection; cleanse and reassess for odor
Tips	• If surrounding skin is very fragile a hydrocolloid is inadvisable due to self-adhesive properties • Hypergranulation can occur under these dressings—observe for this complication • Best applied at room temperature—press the dressing in place with your hand for one minute after applying to improve adherence • Be careful with dressing removal to avoid skin stripping—apply skin sealant before dressing application and remove dressing in the direction of hair growth • If dressing was cut prior to applying, after application, place tape on the cut edge to minimize rolling

Hydrofiber

Hydrofibers are absorptive primary dressings that look like soft fibrous sheets (see Figure 8.10). Hydrofibers are available in pad or ribbon form. When the dressing comes into contact with the wound exudates, it converts to a solid gel and remains in that gel-state, which makes removal easier. It is unique in its absorption characteristics—it wicks drainage vertically, unlike other absorptive dressings. The vertical maceration minimizes peri-wound maceration.

FIGURE 8.10	Hydrofiber Dressings
Indications	• Heavily draining wounds • Low to moderate draining wounds with less frequent dressing changes
Points to ponder/ precautions	• Not for dry or minimally draining wound—will dehydrate the wound
Tips	• These can be helpful under hydrocolloids to allow some absorption—pad lies flat under secondary dressing • When used with depth, place loosely in wound

Other specialty dressings

The following is a list of other specialty dressings available today:

- **Odor-absorbing dressings** contain a layer of activated charcoal to absorb exudate and neutralize the odor. They are used primarily for moderately draining wounds. These dressings are good choices when wound odor is a problem or wound drainage affects quality of life.

- **Antimicrobial dressings** provide an antimicrobial barrier to the wound. Although these dressings reduce the bioburden of the wound and absorb exudate, they do not cure infections. *Be sure to read product information very carefully—some silver dressings should be activated with sterile water instead of saline because saline will precipitate the silver as silver chloride.*

Antimicrobial dressings include the silver dressings and the cadexomer iodine dressings. One type of silver dressing has tiny crystals of silver, copper, and zinc that release silver ions into the wound when the crystals are broken down by adding water. One benefit of silver dressings is the stable and consistent release of silver ions to the wound bed, as opposed to the high and low concentrations that can occur with topical silver products. Cadexomer iodine dressings also have proven to be effective without causing the concern for iodine toxicity associated with povidone iodine. The cadexomer iodine dressings are absorptive and slowly release the iodine.

- **Growth factors** are not actually a dressing but are topical treatments that cause certain cells to proliferate or migrate. Different growth factors target different cells. In practice, these growth factors tend to be used most often for diabetic ulcers than for pressure ulcers.

Adjuvant wound therapy

When conventional wound care does not result in progress of healing the wound, consider adjuvant therapies. These therapies are conducted in conjunction with topical wound management. Examples include electrical stimulation, negative pressure wound therapy (NPWT), and hyperbaric oxygen.

Electrical stimulation

The Agency for Healthcare Research and Quality guidelines support use of electrical stimulation for treatment of chronic pressure ulcers that have not responded to conventional treatment. The stimulation is based on the influence of electrical charge—both positive and negative polarity—on wound healing. Several properly designed, randomized controlled studies have been conducted, and the strength of evidence supporting its use has been upgraded to the highest rating. In one study, electrical stimulation resulted in a 43% increase in the healing rate of pressure ulcers.[1]

The electrical current has a stimulatory effect on fibroblasts and collagen synthesis. This stimulation is believed to improve blood flow and reduce the load of microorganisms known to live in chronic wounds. Physical therapists usually provide this therapy.

Negative pressure wound therapy

NPWT is also known as vacuum-assisted closure. This therapy involves exposing a wound to subatmospheric pressure. The concept converts an open wound to a controlled, closed wound while removing excess fluid from the wound bed, thus increasing circulation/disposal of cellular waste.

Clinical benefits include increased blood flow, decreased bacterial colonization, the ability to quantify the amount of exudate, and increased rate of granulation. It can be used for a variety of wounds but is contraindicated if there is necrotic tissue, untreated osteomyelitis, fistulas, or malignancy. It is also contraindicated if the dressing would be directly over exposed arteries or veins in the wound. *Note:* Use caution with NPWT if the patient is on anticoagulation therapy.

A thorough assessment of the patient should be performed before initiation of NPWT. Some factors to consider are the patient's nutritional status (albumin/prealbumin levels), diabetes control, systemic steroid, immunosuppression, and patient compliance with dressing regimes.

If you plan to use NPWT, have the device representative train you to ensure proper use of the equipment and dressings and appropriate settings for therapy.

In NPWT, a transparent dressing is placed over the wound. When therapy is initiated, you should visualize the dressing contract down and become tight to indicate an airtight seal. Typically, change the dressing every 48 hours, and record the amount of wound drainage each shift or according to hospital policy. Dressing changes can be painful, so remember to assess your patient and provide analgesics as ordered to address procedural pain.

Hyperbaric oxygen

Additional research is being conducted to determine the therapeutic effectiveness of hyperbaric oxygen (HBO) for pressure ulcers. HBO increases the oxygen-carrying capacity of blood so that it can deliver more oxygen to the tissues.

Note that there are numerous contraindicated diagnoses that may make it only marginally useful for or available to your patients. A prime consideration for this focuses on the etiology of wound hypoxia. If hypoxia is due to pressure, then pressure relief is needed but not necessarily via HBO. On the other hand, if a limb is hypoxic due to little or no circulation, maximizing oxygen to the wound may help salvage a limb. HBO is a very expensive adjuvant therapy.

Surgical options

If it is appropriate, the AHCPR Guidelines recommend use of the most effective and least traumatic method to repair the ulcer. Techniques used include direct closure, skin grafts, skin flaps, and musculocutaneous and free flaps. Minimize pressure to the operative site by using specialty support surfaces. Caregiver education regarding skin inspection and pressure reduction is important to help prevent recurrence.

How does wound therapy history affect future therapies?

Knowledge of wound therapies, available products, and research on this topic changes every day. Some of the therapies undergoing research include phototherapy, topical estrogen patches, and topical phenytoin. Advances in biotechnology are amazing, but overall, healthcare professionals are probably not as enlightened to wound management processes as they should be, as illustrated by the fact that moist wound healing has been validated since the 1960s but a 1994 study of home healthcare nurses reported dry gauze the dressing of choice 77% of the time. Therefore, continually update your knowledge of wound therapies and be sure to care for your patients using established principles and practices of wound management.

Next steps

Once your initial assessments are completed and you have chosen a wound cleansing method and a topical treatment/dressing, develop interventions based on all the assessments you conducted. Initiate pain management programs if necessary and continually reassess them to confirm their effectiveness. Conduct a medical evaluation to identify and address diagnoses that affect pressure ulcer development and healing. Confirm that either the treating physician or the nurse practitioner reviewed medications, with special emphasis on those that may impair healing—e.g., corticosteroids, nonsteroidal antiinflammatories, and chemotherapeutic agents.

Once you have assessed the pressure ulcer, the physician has conducted a medical evaluation, and you have chosen a topical wound product/dressing, make sure you have done the following:

- Implemented positioning strategies and devices
- Identified support surfaces for the wheelchair and bed
- Ensured rehabilitative services are provided, if needed
- Created a management plan for incontinence
- Created a nutritional plan to support wound healing and to address nutritional deficiencies

References

1. Gardner, S.E., R.A. Frantz, and F.L. Schmidt. 1999. Effect of electrical stimulation on chronic wound healing: A meta-analysis. *Wound Repair and Regeneration* 7: 495–503.

Wound Healing

"Healing is a matter of time, but it is sometimes also a matter of opportunity."

—Hippocrates

As the above quote suggests, conduct regular and systematic wound assessments, and seize every opportunity to improve your patient's potential to heal. Wound assessment and management is only fractionally addressed by selecting the most effective topical treatment. If you try only to manage the pressure ulcer, you cheat your patient of the collective wisdom of the team and will be unable to ensure the most effective outcomes possible.

There is a theme here that you must embrace: Pressure ulcer prevention and management are multi-faceted and cannot be conducted in a bubble. Assessment of wound healing requires the same interdisciplinary approach. Although dimensions are very important descriptors, assessment cannot be conducted by measurement alone. All of the components of assessment outlined in this book are important to your subsequent assessments.

The standard of practice requires *at least* weekly measurement of the wound. In addition, every time you change the dressing, assess peri-wound skin, wound margins, wound tissue, drainage, odor, pain, and any other relevant issues. On a weekly basis, assess those macroscopic (i.e., visible to the naked eye) indices, measure the wound, assess the effectiveness of the treatment, and determine any treatment plan changes.

Is it healing?

It may be difficult for you to determine whether a wound is improving or whether it needs a change in the topical-treatment approach. As pressure ulcers heal, they may change shape or dimension, making this part of the job even more difficult. For example, what does it mean when one measurement improves and the other declines? An objective tool can help you determine a patient's progress toward healing and eliminate the need for personal opinions or interpretation.

The Pressure Ulcer Scale for Healing (PUSH) Tool (see Figure 9.1) is one such objective—and research-validated—tool. The National Pressure Ulcer Advisory Panel (NPUAP) developed it, and many experts strongly advocate its use—it is easy and reliable. The PUSH Tool is designed to monitor the three parameters that are most indicative of healing:

- Length x width—scored 0 to 10, based on the measurements obtained
- Exudate amount—scored 0 (none) to 3 (heavy)
- Tissue type—scored 0 (closed) to 4 (necrotic tissue)

Each characteristic is assigned a numerical score, and the three subscores are added to obtain the total score. This total score is then placed on a pressure-ulcer–healing graph (part of the tool), which makes it easy to determine whether the wound is progressing, staying the same, or deteriorating over time. If the wound is healing, the score will decrease. If the wound is deteriorating, the score will increase.

The following is an example of how this objective tool can affect your practice. For a patient with a 100% necrotic pressure ulcer that has light drainage and measures 2.1 cm x 2.2 cm, make the following calculations:

- 2.1 cm x 2.2 cm: Multiply the two numbers for a total of 4.62. When correlated with the PUSH tool, it would score as a 7.
- Light drainage is scored as 1.
- 100% necrotic tissue type is scored as 4 (it is scored as 4 if there is any amount of necrotic eschar).
- Total PUSH score = 12.

FIGURE 9.1 **PUSH Tool 3.0**

Patient name: _____ Patient ID#:: _____

Ulcer location:_____ Date: _____

DIRECTIONS:

Observe and measure the pressure ulcer. Categorize the ulcer with respect to surface area, exudate, and type of wound tissue. Record a subscore for each of these ulcer characteristics. Add the subscores to obtain the total score. A comparison of total scores measured over time provides an indication of the improvement or deterioration in pressure ulcer healing.

Length	0	1	2	3	4	5	
	0 cm^2	$< 0.3 \text{ cm}^2$	$0.3\text{-}0.6 \text{ cm}^2$	$0.7\text{-}1.0 \text{ cm}^2$	$1.1\text{-}2.0 \text{ cm}^2$	$2.1\text{-}3.0 \text{ cm}^2$	
x **Width**		6	7	8	9	10	**Subscore**
		$3.1\text{-} 4.0 \text{ cm}^2$	$4.1\text{-}8.0 \text{ cm}^2$	$8.1\text{-}12.0 \text{ cm}^2$	$12.1\text{-}24.0 \text{ cm}^2$	$>24.0 \text{ cm}^2$	
Exudate amount	0	1	2	3			**Subscore**
	None	Light	Moderate	Heavy			
Tissue type	0	1	2	3	4		**Subscore**
	Closed	Epithelial tissue	Granulation tissue	Slough	Necrotic tissue		
							Total score

Length x width: Measure the greatest length (head to toe) and the greatest width (side to side) using a centimeter ruler. Multiply these two measurements (length x width) to obtain an estimate of surface area in square centimeters (cm^2). Caveat: Do not guess! Always use a centimeter ruler, and always use the same method each time the ulcer is measured.

Exudate amount: Estimate the amount of exudate (drainage) present after removal of the dressing and before applying any topical agent to the ulcer. Estimate the exudate (drainage) as none, light, moderate, or heavy.

Tissue type: This refers to the types of tissue that are present in the wound (ulcer) bed. Score as a "4" if there is any necrotic tissue present.   Score as a "3" if there is any amount of slough present and necrotic tissue is absent. Score as a "2" if the wound is clean and contains granulation tissue. A superficial wound that is reepithelializing is scored as a "1." When the wound is closed, score as a "0."

   4 – **Necrotic tissue (Eschar):** black, brown, or tan tissue that adheres firmly to the wound bed or ulcer edges and may be either firmer or softer than surrounding skin.
   3 – **Slough:** yellow or white tissue that adheres to the ulcer bed in strings or thick clump, or is mucinous.
   2 – **Granulation tissue**: pink or beefy red tissue with a shiny, moist, granular appearance.
   1 – **Epithelial tissue:** for superficial ulcers or new pink, or shiny tissue (skin) that grows in from the edges or as islands on the ulcer surface.
   0 – **Closed/resurfaced:** the wound is completely covered with epithelium (new skin).

FIGURE 9.1

PUSH Tool 3.0 (cont.)

PRESSURE ULCER HEALING CHART
(To monitor trends in PUSH scores over time)
(Use a separate page for each pressure ulcer)

Patient name: _____ Patient ID#:: _____

Ulcer location: _____ Date: _____

DIRECTIONS:
Observe and measure pressure ulcers at regular intervals using the PUSH Tool. Date and record PUSH subscale and total scores on the pressure ulcer healing record below.

	PRESSURE ULCER HEALING RECORD
DATE	
Length x width	
Exudate amount	
Tissue type	
Total score	

Graph the PUSH total score on the pressure ulcer healing graph below.

PUSH Total score	PRESSURE ULCER HEALING GRAPH
17	
16	
15	
14	
13	
12	
11	
10	
9	
8	
7	
6	
5	
4	
3	
2	
1	
Healed 0	
DATE	

FIGURE 9.1

PUSH Tool 3.0 (cont.)

Instructions for sing the PUSH Tool

To use the PUSH Tool, the pressure ulcer is assessed and scored on the three elements in the tool:

- **Length x width** ⟶ scored from 0 to 10
- **Exudate amount** ⟶ scored from 0 (none) to 3 (heavy)
- **Tissue type** ⟶ scored from 0 (closed) to 4 (necrotic tissue)

In order to ensure consistency in applying the tool to monitor wound healing, definitions for each element are supplied at the bottom of the tool.

Step 1: Using the definition for length x width, a centimeter ruler measurement is made of the greatest head-to-toe diameter. A second measurement is made of the greatest width (left to right). Multiple these two measurements to get square centimeters and then select the corresponding category for size on the scale and record the score.

Step 2: Estimate the amount of exudate after removal of the dressing and before applying any topical agents. Select the corresponding category for amount, and record the score.

Step 3: Identify the type of tissue. Note: If there is ANY necrotic tissue, it is scored as a 4. Or, if there is ANY slough, it is scored as a 3, even though most of the wound is covered with granulation tissue.

Step 4: Sum the scores on the three elements of the tool to derive a total PUSH Score.

Step 5: Transfer the total score to the Pressure Ulcer Healing Graph. Changes in the score over time provide an indication of the changing status of the ulcer. If the score goes down, the wound is healing. If it gets larger, the wound is deteriorating.

PUSH Tool Version 3.0: 9/15/98
Source: Used with permission of the National Pressure Ulcer Advisory Panel. This tool is not to be used for proprietary presentations and courses.

When you reassess the wound one week later, the necrosis is gone, and there is granulation tissue throughout the wound bed with light drainage—but length x width measurements have increased to 2.7 cm x 2.4 cm. Score as follows:

- 2.7 cm x 2.4 cm: Multiplied, this equals 6.48, and when correlated with the PUSH Tool it is scored as 7.
- Light drainage is scored as 1.
- 100% granulation tissue is scored as 2.
- Total PUSH score = 10.

So, has the wound improved? Yes. Although the length and width measurements have increased, the pressure ulcer has improved because there is now healthy granulation tissue. This is important to understand. Too frequently, nurses document wounds as having deteriorated solely based on measurements.

In the case of wound depth, similar issues arise. If the wound base is covered with slough, for instance, the true depth of the wound is difficult to determine. You can obtain measurements, but expect the depth to increase when you eradicate the slough. As in the previous example, this increase does not represent deterioration even though it may seem to do so.

If your hospital does not use the PUSH Tool or some form of objective measurement, be especially careful about the conclusions you reach regarding pressure ulcer progress.

Monitoring healing

Pressure-ulcer–healing rates are based on so many different factors that it is difficult to predict how long they take to heal. In addition, the age of the wound affects healing rates, and some chronic wounds may never heal. The following is a very general guideline for healing rates:

- Stage I—one day to one week
- Stage II—five days to three months
- Stage III—one month to six months
- Stage IV—six months to one year

Expect chronic wounds to be your biggest challenge—they result from complications that delay wound healing, and disruption of the normal flow of blood is common to all of them. They may only show 0.5

cm improvement in one month, which could be considered satisfactory progress for such a wound. Because chronic wounds are often associated with such miniscule progress, you must use accurate measurement techniques, or you may not detect any progress.

What about wounds that are at a definite standstill? They could be either slow-to-respond chronic wounds or wounds that, despite alternative treatment, have not changed in any way. Pressure ulcers should show movement toward healing within two to four weeks of treatment. If they have not responded at that point, revise your treatment approach. If the wound deteriorates, change the treatment at the time that you detect deterioration. The AHRQ and the Wound, Ostomy and Continence Nurses Society pressure ulcer guidelines advise consideration of a two-week trial of topical antibiotics for pressure ulcers that are not healing or are continuing to produce exudates after two to four weeks of optimal care.

Recalcitrant wounds

Wounds that have been appropriately and comprehensively managed typically show progress within two to four weeks. If they do not progress during that period, they may be labeled "recalcitrant," or resistant to treatment. The emphasis here is not necessarily on the time factor but rather on the appropriate and comprehensive management, in addition to the time factor. Some believe that all wounds should show improvement in two to four weeks, but do not just go by that time interval—you need to be sure that during that time there was proper overall management as well. A great topical treatment for two weeks may not yield progress without pressure relief.

What does appropriate and comprehensive management look like? It includes many of the factors discussed throughout this book, including the following:

- Correction or alleviation of causative factors
- System support, including management of disease and nutritional support
- Adherence to principles of wound management, including maintenance of a clean, moist wound; control of bioburden of the wound; elimination of necrotic tissue; and filling of dead space

If all of the above factors have been consistently addressed for four weeks, and the pressure ulcer fails to make any progress, consider it recalcitrant. Investigate further to determine why healing has not progressed. Perhaps different nutritional support is needed or the bioburden of the wound is heavy (this refers to the heavy "load" of microorganisms in the wound) without showing visible signs of infection. Sometimes you will not be able to determine the reason the wound is recalcitrant, but your documentation should reflect the interventions and your analysis. When managing a recalcitrant wound, adjuvant treatments may be an option.

There is a difference between a recalcitrant wound and one that simply becomes unresponsive to a particular treatment. You will find pressure ulcers that respond to the topical treatment for several weeks and then all of a sudden stop making progress. Often a simple change in type of topical treatment "wakes up" the wound and it begins to respond again. Remember, when making such changes, adhere to the general principles of wound management.

Different treatments (like different shampoos for hair) interact with the wound in distinct manners. They are manufactured differently and may have different surfactants. One is not necessarily better than the other, but because it is different, it may cause the wound to stand up and take notice.

What happens when you close a pressure ulcer?

Proceed with caution with a newly closed pressure ulcer. Although your inclination may be to "resolve" or end the pressure ulcer care plan, doing so would be unwise. A closed wound will never be normal in structure or function. After a year of remodeling, the tissue will only have approximately 75% of its original tensile strength and will remain weakened. Minimizing the risk of recurrence will be a lifelong struggle.

The NPUAP position statement, "The Facts about Reverse Staging in 2000," states, "If a pressure ulcer reopens in the same anatomical site, the ulcer resumes the previous staging diagnosis (i.e., once a Stage IV, always a Stage IV)." Recurrence rates in adults for pressure ulcers at the same site reportedly range from 13%–56%. Therefore, be vigilant in monitoring for recurrence of pressure ulcers, and maintain strong preventive practices.

Even if you address risk management for patients, also manage the hospital's risk by educating the patient's family. In the case of a closed pressure ulcer, inform the patient and the family of the potential for recurrence. Advise them that if the pressure ulcer were to reopen, it would return to its prior stage. No one likes this kind of surprise, and although you hope to prevent recurrence, it may happen. If you provide the patient and family with a thorough explanation, they will be less likely to perceive recurrence as a failure in the care your hospital provided.

Common Treatment and Documentation Problems

This discussion of wound healing would not be complete without a mention of the common problems observed in many organizations. It's difficult to determine a treatment's effectiveness, for example, if it is not being administered in the way it was ordered. Nurses should never take creative liberties with physician-ordered treatments.

For the most part, offending nurses really do not even understand that they are doing anything wrong when, for example, they substitute a secondary dressing. But conducting any treatment not as ordered is the same as committing a medication error, and it should be documented similarly. A "laissez-faire" approach to substitutions, omissions, or changes made without physician orders will result in less successful outcomes for your patients. As it is a risk-management issue for both the patient and the facility, you must take any such tendency in your hospital seriously.

Follow treatments as ordered

Often, however, organizations take a casual stance on treatment administration. Nurses at change of shift (usually between first and second) can often be overheard saying, "I didn't get a chance to do treatments on that side, so if you can get to them that would be good." Such a request should raise red flags for your hospital—how can staff think it's appropriate for a treatment ordered twice a day to be performed only once a day? It would surely raise some eyebrows if you heard a nurse say, "Gee, I was unable to get the noon medications passed, but I knew you'd be passing meds again at 4 p.m., so can you give the noon meds out, too?" Treatments are ordered in specific ways and with specific frequencies. Failing to follow them as ordered is an omission of physician-ordered care and violates nursing-practice standards.

In another common problematic scenario, a nurse who doesn't agree with the treatment ordered substitutes a different product. Indeed, nurses often use a different treatment at bedside than was ordered but would not dream of substituting a different medication without first addressing any concerns with the physician. Why are wound treatments a different story? Take these matters seriously. The practice of such casual substitution is both frustrating and poor.

If you are faced with not having the appropriate supplies available to conduct the treatment, which of the following should you do?

    a) Circle your initials and write on the back of the treatment sheet "not available"
    b) Leave the treatment sheet blank because you can't do it
    c) Call the physician and ask for a substitute order, using a product that is available in house, until the other product becomes available

The obvious answer is "c," but an oft-noted practice is "a." One possible solution to the problem is to develop a house protocol, approved by your director of nurses and medical director, that addresses the issue of unavailable products/supplies. This protocol should serve as a temporary intervention to allow some form of treatment while the prescribed product is unavailable.

The following is an example of language for such a protocol: "If at any time a topical product is not available for pressure ulcer treatment, a normal saline wet-to-moist dressing may be applied for the ordered treatment frequency, for a 24-hour period." This should give you enough time to obtain products you need to resume the previously ordered treatment. Remember, you would need to transcribe the protocol when it is put in place and follow the other hospital procedures outlined, such as physician notification, if required.

One last word of caution regarding documentation on treatment records, involving the words "as above" and "treatment done as ordered": There are cases in which nurses document "as above" if their assessment of the wound was the same as the prior description on the treatment sheet. Doing so is not good practice, and it could be questioned if the chart ever came under legal scrutiny. Instead, provide specifically your assessment of the wound, including the amount of drainage on the dressing you removed. Simply writing "as above" is tantamount to saying you couldn't be bothered to write your own assessment.

As a licensed nurse, you understand your obligation to assess the wound and to write your assessment on the treatment sheet (or to use the appropriate form of documentation your hospital uses). Writing "treatment done as ordered" may fill the spot for that shift's documentation, but that phrase is not a wound description. Note that it is also good practice to date, time, and initial every dressing you apply.

Care planning

Problems described in patient care plans must be thorough and descriptive. A care plan problem that states, "At risk for pressure ulcer development due to immobility and incontinence" is unoriginal and incomplete. The "problem" area of the care plan needs to identify all the risks to ensure that you assess all the individual factors that place a patient at risk or that must be considered in treatment of an actual pressure ulcer. Figure 10.1 is a partial list of such risk factors—and the reasons for their importance.

Next, the interdisciplinary team needs to determine the goal of a patient's treatment. For an at-risk patient, the goal is typically prevention. For a patient with a pressure-related injury that has already occurred, decide whether the goal is healing, maintenance, or comfort. Further define your goals by determining the following:

- If you can improve the problem (pressure ulcer), develop a specific and measurable goal that is realistic. For example,
    - "pressure ulcer will be free of necrotic tissue within 30 days"
    - "pressure ulcer will reduce in size by 1 cm within 30 days"
- If you cannot improve the pressure ulcer, the goal should be to prevent or minimize complications or decline. For example,
    - "pressure ulcer will be free of signs and symptoms of infection for 30 days"
    - "pressure ulcer will not increase in size (l x w x d) in next 30 days"
- If pressure ulcer deterioration is inevitable, the goal should be to provide comfort and optimal quality of life within the limitations of the disease process, patient advance-care directives, and patient preferences. For example,
    - "patient's self-reported pain level will be managed at the 0–2 level daily for 30 days"
    - "patient will not detect non-procedure–related wound odor daily for 30 days"

Unlimited interventions

Interventions will arise naturally as you review each risk factor or problem, and they will be guided by the overall goals of care. Potential interventions are unlimited but should be based on the unique needs of each patient. If you use standardized care plans and approaches, remember that they are starting points for care and do not function as an all-inclusive plans.

	Partial List of Care-Plan Risk Factors

FIGURE 10.1

Sample risk factors	How does it affect risk or healing?
Contracture of left lower extremity	• This poses positioning difficulty depending on the degree of the contracture • Blood supply may be impaired (depending on contracture severity), which may result in an ischemic limb at higher risk of pressure ulcer development or delayed healing
Poor intake, low albumin or prealbumin level, weight loss	• Poor nutrition is associated with pressure ulcer development and impaired healing
Limited turning surfaces due to presence of pressure ulcers on left and right trochanter	• Repositioning techniques are limited due to the presence of pressure ulcers on two of four turning surfaces
Head of bed elevation at all times due to acute congestive heart failure	• Head of bed elevation is known to cause shear tissue injury
Pain	• Pain causes vasoconstriction which impairs circulation • Pain will likely result in suboptimal compliance with movement
Diabetes	• Impaired immune function • Loss of lean body mass that is replaced with inactive fat mass • Increased blood glucose impairs blood flow through small vessels • Impairs red blood cell permeability and flow
Immobility	• Sustained pressure causes tissue ischemia • Spinal cord injured—may be capable of moving when desired but doesn't get sensation of when it is time to move (i.e., discomfort)
Anemia	• Poor perfusion of tissues especially if hematocrit drops below 20%
Depression	• May effect level of mobility and appetite
Systemic corticosteroids	• Interfere with regeneration of the epidermis and collagen synthesis
Nonsteroidal anti-inflammatory durgs (NSAID)	• Alter inflammatory reactions
Hematologic abnormalities	• Impaired healing with WBC deficiencies • Reduction in RBCs delays healing due to less oxygen delivery
Edema	• Edematous tissue is more prone to breakdown • Impairs circulation by pressure on vessels by accumulation of fluid in tissue spaces • May be an indicator of protein malnutrition
Hypotension	• Associated with impaired blood perfusion to tissue

The basic point is that you must create realistic care plans. The goal needs to be attainable within the context of the patient's clinical realities and preferences, and if you are in the habit of writing "Pressure ulcer will heal by next review," you need to change that habit.

Developing a thorough care plan gives you a great starting point, but communicating the plan and putting it into practice is an even bigger task. This process varies from organization to organization, but in all cases, direct caregivers must be aware of their responsibilities. Therefore, there has to be a reliable system in place that relays the information to those responsible for that aspect of care. For example, nursing assistants, or nursing technicians, have enormous responsibilities and often are left uninformed—but are held accountable for—the aspects of care that are most important to the patient. Evaluate the strengths and weaknesses of your current communication systems with a focus on how to convey new needs or revised interventions (see Chapter 11 for examples of tools to use to assess your pressure ulcer program).

Often, it is not until you feel the enormity of the task that you realize one policy and one person cannot do it alone. The pressure ulcer problem has far-reaching effects, and correcting it takes the talents of an entire team. A multitude of studies have shown the positive difference in outcomes that involve well-established teams.

Wound-care experts generally agree that the wound-care team is the strongest determinant of your program's success. Important elements of the team include member education, enthusiasm for the task, tools used, outcomes measured, and patient perceptions of the program.

Education

Education is a key component of effective pressure ulcer prevention and treatment programs. In addition to educating wound-care team members, instruct primary caregivers, patients, families, and other professional staff on all aspects of risk and care, including but not limited to the following:

- Risk factors for pressure ulcer development
- Routine skin assessment
- Support surfaces
- Positioning principles
- Continence and incontinence management
- Care-plan development and implementation
- Documentation systems
- Hospital systems, guidelines, and protocols

Pressure ulcer education is sometimes conducted during orientation of new staff, but generally it is not provided as routinely or comprehensively as it should be. And while we often complain about regulatory scrutiny—such as that related to incomplete pressure ulcer care—note regulatory priorities. For example, when it comes to fire regulations, annual training is required, as are monthly drills and standard equipment and fire-management systems. The purpose of extensive fire-safety regulations is not to make more work for staff; rather, it is to protect patients. The same is true of pressure ulcer education.

Most elderly patients face the daily risk of pressure ulcer development. Pressure ulcers cost more than $1 billion per year to treat, affect quality of life, result in morbidity and mortality, and lead to a continual rise in lawsuits with exorbitant settlements.

Hospital commitment and values set the stage for all subsequent work, attitudes, and systems. Therefore, ask how your organization conveys them as they relate to pressure ulcer prevention, assessment, and treatment. Articulate your hospital's values and expectations with a concurrent commitment of human and fiscal resources:

- ✔ Clearly state your hospital's intent to avoid all pressure ulcers by applying a rigorous prevention and treatment program based on accepted standards of practice.

- ✔ Use accepted standards of practice to develop meaningful, hospital-based policies, procedures, and protocols.

- ✔ Establish accountability for the program—the who, what, when, where, and how.

- ✔ Provide needed equipment and staff to support the goals—with pressure ulcers, you often reap what you sow. Staff cannot truly pursue a goal of pressure ulcer prevention if there is insufficient staffing and no money for prevention products (e.g., incontinence care products, pressure-relieving devices, etc.).

- ✔ Make education a top priority. Regularly educate all levels of staff, patients, and families.

- ✔ Put in place a plan for evaluation and reevaluation of your program with an expectation of continuous quality improvement.

- ✔ Proclaim your successes. Sometimes you get so caught up in what has not been done correctly that you forget to enjoy the mini-successes along the way.

- ✔ Share the program's progress and success with staff to prove leadership's attention and sustained commitment to pressure ulcer prevention, assessment, and treatment.

Risk management

It is not fear of legal issues that should motivate you but rather patients' dependence on you to care for them. Nevertheless, note that when prevention and treatment of pressure ulcers comes under legal scrutiny, it is often alleged as negligence. Pressure ulcer negligence suits differ from others in one substantive way: They are not usually based on one incident. As a comparison, look at a fall lawsuit—although it requires risk assessment, care planning, and provision of interventions, it is often a failure on one day (resulting in a fall with injury) that is the basis of the negligence charge. Pressure ulcers, however, develop over time, and time is needed to treat the pressure ulcer; thus, the plaintiff (usually a family member) and his or her attorney look for patterns in the clinical record. Even if great care was provided, you will not be able to prove it if documentation does not reflect thorough assessment and care consistent with standards of practice.

If your pressure ulcer prevention and management practices come under scrutiny, consider these three very important factors:

1. The medical record must reflect strict adherence to the standard of care for pressure ulcers

2. The medical record must contain documentation of patient complications, risk factors underlying diseases that made the development of pressure ulcers unavoidable

3. Provide a comprehensive and aggressive program to prevent and treat the pressure ulcer (within the confines of the patient's care directives)

Develop a team approach to preventing/treating pressure ulcers that includes the patient and his or her family. When your education efforts help a patient and family know and understand all the steps of care and when they have participated in the treatment plan, they are less inclined to find blame or seek legal retribution.

When you have a systems approach that is based on accepted standards of practice and is consistently followed, you will know that you have done everything possible to prevent pressure ulcers. In addition, you should now understand how to assess, document, and treat those ulcers you are unable to prevent.

Avoidable v. unavoidable pressure ulcers

Some experts believe that all pressure ulcers are avoidable. Others believe that there are times when the patient's risk factors or deterioration of health is so significant that even the best preventive care could not thwart pressure ulcer development. Such a situation, however, is the exception, not the rule.

Often, a review of the patient's hospital stay can give insight to whether a pressure ulcer could have been avoided. Was there a risk assessment performed and, if the patient was deemed at-risk, were protocols initiated? Was there a change in the patient's status that warranted a revision of the protocol? Were interventions carried out and documented consistently? Answering these questions provides valuable information for the multidisciplinary team.

Assessment tools

Use quality assessment tools to document your findings and ensure that you are giving optimum care to patients with pressure ulcers. They help you identify and manage patient and facility risks and will result in better outcomes.

Use the tools given in this chapter (see Figures 11.1–11.5) to assess your pressure ulcer systems. Some tools are generic and may need to be revised to reflect the specific details within your hospital. Permission is not needed to use these forms in your hospital.

| FIGURE 11.1 | **Quality Assessment/Improvement Tool** |

Patient Name:_____   Rm#:_____

UNAVOIDABLE PRESSURE ULCER(S)—QA/QI REVIEW

The patient has and continues to receive all necessary care and services to attain/maintain the highest practicable physical, mental, and psychosocial well-being in accordance with the patient's individual assessment and plan of care. The patient's medical diagnosis and complicating factors leads us to conclude the patient's pressure ulcer(s) are unavoidable.

The patient's pressure ulcer(s) are unavoidable because the patient has impaired mobility and two (2) or more of the following clinical conditions:

❏ Severe COPD   ❏ Diabetes   ❏ Severe Peripheral Vascular Disease
❏ Sepsis   ❏ Bowel Incontinence   ❏ Continuous urinary Incontinence
❏ Paraplegia   ❏ Quadriplegia   ❏ Body Cast
❏ Terminal Cancer   ❏ Immunosuppression   ❏ Chronic liver, renal and/or heart disease
          ❏ Malnutrition or Failure to Thrive:
                    ❏ Serum albumin below 3.4 g/dl or Prealbumin below 15 mg/dl
                    ❏ Serum transferring level below 180 mg/dl
                    ❏ Hemoglobin less than 12 mg/dl
                    ❏ Poor skin turgor
                    ❏ Reduced urinary output
                    ❏ Weight loss of more than 10% during the past month
                    ❏ Bilateral edema
                    ❏ Muscle wasting
The patient receives two (2) or more of the following treatments:
          ❏ Steroid Therapy   ❏ Radiation Therapy   ❏ Chemotherapy
          ❏ Renal Dialysis   ❏ HOB elevated due to medical necessity
❏ The patient is terminally ill, semi-comatose, or comatose, and life-sustaining measures have been withdrawn
❏ The patient has a prior history of pressure ulcers in the same location

Other clinical conditions/issues/risk factors:
_____
_____

The following interventions were put into place to address risk factors and clinical conditions:_____
_____
_____

The following patient/family education was
provided:_____
_____

Quality Review Conducted by:
Signatures: _____   Date:_____
           _____   Date:_____
           _____   Date:_____
           _____   Date:_____

FIGURE 11.2 — New Pressure Ulcer Checklist

Patient Name:_____ Date:_____

When a new pressure ulcer is noted you must set several things into action. Please use this checklist as a guideline to be sure the patient receives all the needed services and support.

Assess

❏ Conduct initial assessment and fill in on the _____ form

- Location and stage
- Measurements (length X width X depth), measure tunnels or undermining with "cm" and location of tunnel and undermining (according to clock)
- Exudate (color and amount), odor (determine after cleaning wound)
- Wound-base tissue description—epithelial tissue, granulation, slough, eschar—in %
- Peri-wound tissue description
- Any pain assessed or reported

❏ Assess chair and bed surface for pressure relief devices on or needed

❏ If pressure ulcer on heel/foot—discuss discontinuing use of leather footwear/sneakers

Notifications

❏ Notify physician and obtain orders—as appropriate

- for localized care
- pain management
- consultations—rehab, dietary, other
- specialty bed if needed
- lab work—Hgb, Hct, Albumin or Prealbumin, BUN, Creatinine
- Vitamin support—Multivitamin with minerals, Vitamin C, Zinc Sulfate (if ordered, suggest only 2–4 weeks)

❏ Notify patient and family/responsible person of pressure ulcer and onset of treatment plan

❏ Notify nursing assistant via _____ (Collaborate with Nursing Assistant/Technician regarding treatment plan)

❏ Notify Registered Dietitian to obtain nutritional assessment

❏ Notify _____, Wound Team member

❏ Notify Nursing Unit Supervisor/Director of Nurses (or designee) _____ to follow hospital chain of command

❏ Notify P.T. to assess seating cushion, request screen, and/or convey MD order for consultation

❏ Notify pharmacy consultant to assess med regimen for evaluation of meds contributing to risk

Documentation

❏ Transcribe treatment on treatment sheet

❏ Transcribe new physician orders

❏ Initiate pressure ulcer monitoring/measurement tracking form

❏ Initiate PUSH Tool

❏ Initiate repositioning schedule (unless patient is independent)

❏ Initiate pressure ulcer care plan

❏ Comprehensive nurses note (in addition to treatment sheet documentation for new ulcers)

- Full description of pressure ulcer (per the Assessment section)
- Notifications made
- Consults initiated
- Pressure relief devices provided
- New orders
- Assessment of pain (and intervention/effect if pain reported)

FIGURE 11.3	**Wound Assessment Tool**

Patient name:

❏ Pressure   ❏ Other   location:_____

Date:	Initial assessment							
Length (cm.)								
Width (cm.)								
Depth (cm.)								
Stage								
Undermining/tunneling (cm.)								
Wound base								
Ulcer margins								
Exudate								
Odor								
Periwound skin								
Pain								
Pressure reduction interventions 1. Pressure reducing mattress 2. W/C cushion 3. Specialty bed 4. Other_____ _____								
Debridement yes/no type								
PUSH Tool score								
Improved, same, deteriorated								
Treatment appropriate yes/no								
Last change in treatment (date)								
MD notified of change (date)								
Family notified of change (date)								
Nurse's initials								

FIGURE 11.4	Pressure Ulcer Assessment Report							
Wound base								
Peri-wound tissue								
Odor								
Exudate amt. and color								
Under-mining cm and location								
Tunnel cm and location								
Depth (cm)								
Width (cm)								
Length (cm)								
Stage								
Site								
Patient name								
Date								

FIGURE 11.5   Sample Care-Plan Goals

Care-plan goals must be established within the clinical reality of the patient for whom you are care planning. A multitude of care-plan goals may be appropriate, and the following is a partial listing of some indicators of healing that could be incorporated for pressure ulcers with healing potential.

Necrotic wound

- Wound will be free of eschar and necrotic debris within _____ days

- Eschar will decrease is size by 50% within _____ days (current eschar measurement 4 cm x 3 cm)

Infected wound

- Purulent, malodorous wound exudates will be serous or serosanguinous with no odor within _____ days

- Peri-wound skin and wound margins will be free of erythema, edema, and induration within _____ days

Undermining wound

- Undermining of wound will decrease by 0.5 cm within _____ days (current undermining of 4 cm from 2 o'clock to 6 o'clock)

- Wound will be free of undermining and wound margins will attach within _____ days (current undermining of 0.5 cm at 2 o'clock to 4 o'clock)

Clean wound

- Wound will have increased granulation tissue resulting in a reduction of wound depth of 0.5 cm within _____ days

- Wound will be fully granulated within _____ days

- Wound contraction will begin and surface area (length x width) of wound will reduce by 1 cm within _____ days

- Wound will begin to re-epithelialize at wound margins within _____ days

- Wound will be 100% resurfaced with epithelial tissue within _____ days

Target audience:

Staff nurses and nurse managers

Statement of need:

This book approaches nurse-physician communication trouble spots by coupling anecdotal scenarios with tangible advice for nurses. It will offer field-tested, how-to advice for helping nurses fully understand and cope with communication breakdown that often occurs between doctors and nurses. The book will consist of case scenarios, critical-thinking activities, and other tools to help nurses better understand and communicate with their physician counterparts.

Educational objectives:

Upon completion of this activity, participants should be able to do the following:

- Define "pressure ulcer" and explain the role of impaired blood supply in the creation of pressure ulcers
- Identify two influences that put patients at risk for pressure ulcers and that may be beyond the caregivers' control
- Define the "rule of 30," and explain where on the body pressure is prevented by using this rule
- Identify two reasons why heels are the second most common sites of pressure ulcers and provide an example of how to "off-load" pressure from this area
- List and explain the four pressure ulcer stages
- Define "backstaging" and explain why it is not recommended
- Identify the two most widely used risk-assessment tools, and list two of the subscales covered by each tool
- List four intrinsic and extrinsic risk factors for pressure ulcer development
- List and identify the four types of tissue to be observe in a pressure ulcer
- Identify the three-dimensional measurement formula, and list two related measurement techniques

- State three possible strategies nurses can perform to relieve pain during dressing changes
- Identify and differentiate the three possible microbiologic states within pressure ulcers
- Define "MVTR," and identify good and bad MVTR
- List the seven "rights" to consider when performing dressing changes
- List two wound-care products that promote a moist wound environment
- Define "negative pressure wound therapy," and list two factors to consider about the patient before administering this therapy
- Identify and explain the three parameters the PUSH tool is designed to monitor
- List the three factors that must be consistently addressed prior to identifying a wound as "recalcitrant"
- Explain why taking creative liberties with physician-ordered treatments is a bad practice, and give one specific example of this occurrence from your work setting in nursing
- Identify two care-plan risk factors, and explain how they affect risk or healing
- Explain why proper, detailed documentation is important when defending pressure ulcer–related lawsuits
- List three aspects of risk and care about which primary caregivers, patients, families, and other professional staff should be educated

Author:

Karen S. Clay, RN, BSN, CWCN

Accreditation/designation statement:

This educational activity for four contact hours is provided by HCPro, Inc. HCPro is accredited as a provider of continuing nursing education by the American Nurses Credentialing Center's Commission on Accreditation.

Disclosure statements:

Karen S. Clay, Barbara Acello, and Lisa Frizzell have declared that they have no commercial/financial vested interest in this activity.

Instructions

In order to be eligible to receive your nursing contact hour(s) for this activity, you are required to do the following:

1. Read the book
3. Complete the exam
4. Complete the evaluation
5. Provide your contact information in the space provided on the exam and evaluation
6. Submit the exam and evaluation to HCPro, Inc.

Please provide all of the information requested above and mail or fax your completed exam, program evaluation, and contact information to

Robin L. Flynn
Manager, Continuing Education
HCPro, Inc.
200 Hoods Lane
P.O. Box 1168
Marblehead, MA 01945
Fax: 781/639-0179

Nursing education exam

Name: _____

Title: _____

Facility name: _____

Address: _____

Address:

_____

City: _____ State: _____ ZIP: _____

Phone number: _____ Fax number: _____

E-mail: _____

Nursing license number: _____

(ANCC requires a unique identifier for each learner)

1. The Wound, Ostomy and Continence Nurses Society states that a pressure ulcer is any lesion caused by _____.

a. unrelieved pressure   b. undetermined pressure

c. blunt pressure   d. shear

2. According to the text, some experts believe that pressure ulcers are not always preventable. Which of the following influences may be considered beyond the caregivers' control?

a. Patient incontinence   b. Patient malnutrition

c. Patient noncompliance   d. Lack of communication between interdisciplinary team members

3. You are advised to use the "rule of 30" when repositioning patients. This rule instructs you to _____ to prevent pressure over the trochanter and sacrum.

a. elevate the head of the patient's bed every 30 minutes or sooner

b. elevate the head of the patient's bed every 30 seconds or sooner

c. elevate the head of the patient's bed at least 30 times per day

d. elevate the head of the patient's bed to 30° or less

4. Heels have small surface areas and underlying bony surfaces; therefore, redistribution of pressure is nearly impossible. However, _____ is the most effective intervention for removing pressure from, or "off-loading," the heel.

a. elevating the heels with a pillow   b. lying heels flat on the bed

c. using high-density foam blocks   d. using "bunny boots"

5. A _____ pressure ulcer is a wound that involves partial-thickness skin loss involving the epidermis, dermis, or both that presents clinically as an abrasion, a blister, or a shallow crater.

a. Stage I   b. Stage II

c. Stage III   d. Stage IV

6. After a pressure ulcer has healed, the skin's integrity in that area is weaker than that of healthy skin. The healed skin will only have approximately _____ of the tensile strength of undamaged skin.

a. 25%   b. 50%

c. 75%   d. 100%

7. Both the Braden and Norton Scales—pressure ulcer risk-assessment tools—query subsets of information that are assigned numerical ratings, which ultimately determine a patient's risk score/level. Which two subsets are specific to the Norton Scale?

a. Sensory perception and mobiliy   b. Activity and mobility

c. Nutrition and friction and shear   d. Physical and mental condition

8. Intrinsic and extrinsic factors also cause pressure ulcers to develop. Which of the following risk factors is intrinsic?

a. Immobility   b. Friction and shear

c. Moisture   d. Excessive pressure

9. _____ is tissue that contains new blood vessels and connective tissue. It is typically red and moist and often is described by the term "beefy red."

a. Eschar

b. Slough

c. Granulation

d. Epithelial

10. Following the three-dimensional linear wound measuring system, if the measurements for a wound are marked as follows, 4.3 cm x 3.1 cm x 0.9 cm, what do you know is true about the wound?

a. The wound is 3.1 cm long

b. The wound is 3.1 cm deep

c. The wound is 4.3 cm wide

d. The wound is 0.9 cm deep

11. To avoid causing unnecessary pain to patients during dressing changes, always move the _____ away from the _____.

a. tissue; dressing

b. dressing; tissue

c. fingers; dressing

d. tissue; patient

12. Erythema, edema, peri-wound heat, purulent drainage, foul odor, and an increase of pain in the wound are all signs and symptoms of wound _____.

a. contamination

b. colonization

c. infection

d. healing

13. To maintain a moist wound environment, you must achieve a MVTR (moisture vapor transmission rate) of less than _____ grams of water vapor per square meter per hour.

a. 25

b. 35

c. 45

d. 55

14. There are seven correct, or "right," patient or procedure indicators to remember during dressing changes. Which of the following is NOT listed as one of the indicators?

a. Patient

b. Dressing

c. Temperature

d. Time

15. _____ is not recommended because there is concern that it may cause air emboli.

a. Saline

b. Hydrogels

c. Hydrocolloids

d. Hydrogen peroxide

16. _____ involves exposing a wound to subatmospheric pressure to convert the open wound to a controlled, closed wound while removing excess fluid from the wound bed.

a. Hyperbaric oxygen therapy

b. Negative pressure wound therapy

c. Electrical stimulation

d. Surgery

17. The PUSH (Pressure Ulcer Scale for Healing) Tool—developed by the National Pressure Ulcer Advisory Panel—is designed to monitor the three parameters that are most indicative of healing. Which of the following is NOT one of the parameters measured by the tool?

a. Pain

b. Length x width

c. Exudate amount

d. Tissue type

18. If all of the above factors have been consistently addressed for _____ weeks and the pressure ulcer fails to make any progress, consider it "recalcitrant," or resistant to treatment.

a. one

b. two

c. three

d. four

19. If you are faced with not having the appropriate supplies available to conduct a treatment, which of the following should you do?

a. Leave the treatment sheet blank because you can't do it

b. Circle your initials and write on the back of the treatment sheet "not available"

c. Practice "casual substitution" by choosing and applying the order you feel is correct without first speaking to the patient's physician

d. Call the physician and ask for a substitute order, using a product that is available in house, until the other product becomes available

20. _____ is a large risk factor of pressure ulcer development because it impairs the body's immune function, causes increased blood glucose (which impairs blood flow through the small vessels), and impairs red blood cell permeability and flow.

a. Anemia   b. Diabetes

c. Systemic corticosteroids   d. Edema

21. According to the text, pressure ulcers cost more than _____ per year to treat, affect quality of life, result in morbidity and mortality, and lead to a continual rise in lawsuits with exorbitant settlements.

a. $1 billion   b. $2 billion

c. $3 billion   d. $4 billion

22. Routine skin assessments, support surfaces, positioning principles, continence and incontinence management, and care-plan development and implementation are all aspects of pressure ulcer management regarding which many people should receive education. Which of the following groups of people are NOT required to receive education about the aspects of pressure ulcer management listed above?

a. Primary caregivers   b. Patients

c. Families   d. Clergy

Nursing education evaluation

Name: _____

Title: _____

Facility name: _____

Address: _____

Address: _____

City: _____ State: _____ ZIP: _____

Phone number: _____ Fax number: _____

E-mail: _____

Nursing license number: _____

(ANCC requires a unique identifier for each learner)

1. This activity met the following learning objectives:

a.) Define "pressure ulcer" and explain the role of impaired blood supply in the creation of pressure ulcers

    Strongly disagree   1   2   3   4   5   Strongly agree

b.) Identify two influences that put patients at risk for pressure ulcers and that may be beyond the caregivers' control

    Strongly disagree   1   2   3   4   5   Strongly agree

c.) Define the "rule of 30," and explain where on the body pressure is prevented by using this rule

Strongly disagree   1   2   3   4   5   Strongly agree

d.) Identify two reasons why heels are the second most common sites of pressure ulcers and provide an example of how to "off-load" pressure from this area

Strongly disagree   1   2   3   4   5   Strongly agree

e.) List and explain the four pressure ulcer stages

Strongly disagree   1   2   3   4   5   Strongly agree

f.) Define "backstaging" and explain why it is *not* recommended

Strongly disagree   1   2   3   4   5   Strongly agree

g.) Identify the two most widely used risk-assessment tools, and list two of the subscales covered by each tool

Strongly disagree   1   2   3   4   5   Strongly agree

h.) List four intrinsic and extrinsic risk factors for pressure ulcer development

Strongly disagree   1   2   3   4   5   Strongly agree

i.) List and identify the four types of tissue to be observe in a pressure ulcer

Strongly disagree   1   2   3   4   5   Strongly agree

j.) Identify the three-dimensional measurement formula, and list two related measurement techniques

Strongly disagree   1   2   3   4   5   Strongly agree

k.) State three possible strategies nurses can perform to relieve pain during dressing changes

Strongly disagree   1   2   3   4   5   Strongly agree

l.) Identify and differentiate the three possible microbiologic states within pressure ulcers

Strongly disagree   1   2   3   4   5   Strongly agree

m.) Define "MVTR," and identify good and bad MVTR

Strongly disagree   1   2   3   4   5   Strongly agree

n.) List the seven "rights" to consider when performing dressing changes

Strongly disagree   1   2   3   4   5   Strongly agree

o.) List two wound-care products that promote a moist wound environment

Strongly disagree   1   2   3   4   5   Strongly agree

p.) Define "negative pressure wound therapy," and list two factors to consider about the patient before administering this therapy

Strongly disagree   1   2   3   4   5   Strongly agree

q.) Identify and explain the three parameters the PUSH tool is designed to monitor

Strongly disagree   1   2   3   4   5   Strongly agree

r.) List the three factors that must be consistently addressed prior to identifying a wound as "recalcitrant"

Strongly disagree   1   2   3   4   5   Strongly agree

s.) Explain why taking creative liberties with physician-ordered treatments is a bad practice, and give one specific example of this occurrence from your work setting in nursing

Strongly disagree   1   2   3   4   5   Strongly agree

t.) Identify two care-plan risk factors, and explain how they affect risk or healing

Strongly disagree   1   2   3   4   5   Strongly agree

u.) Explain why proper, detailed documentation is important when defending pressure ulcer–related lawsuits

Strongly disagree   1   2   3   4   5   Strongly agree

v.) List three aspects of risk and care about which primary caregivers, patients, families, and other professional staff should be educated

Strongly disagree   1   2   3   4   5   Strongly agree

2. Objectives were related to the overall purpose/goal of the activity

        Strongly disagree   1   2   3   4   5   Strongly agree

3. This activity was related to my nursing activity needs

        Strongly disagree   1   2   3   4   5   Strongly agree

4. The exam for the activity was an accurate test of the knowledge gained

        Strongly disagree   1   2   3   4   5   Strongly agree

5. The activity avoided commercial bias or influence

        Strongly disagree   1   2   3   4   5   Strongly agree

6. This activity met my expectations

        Strongly disagree   1   2   3   4   5   Strongly agree

7. Will this learning activity enhance your professional nursing practice?

    Yes

    No

8. This educational method was an appropriate delivery tool for the nursing/clinical audience

        Strongly disagree   1   2   3   4   5   Strongly agree

9. How committed are you to making the behavioral changes suggested in this activity?

    a) Very committed

    b) Somewhat committed

    c) Not committed

10. Please provide us with your degree

    a) ADN

    b) BSN

    c) MSN

    d) Other, please state

11. Please provide us with your credentials

    a) LVN

    b) LPN

    c) RN

    d) NP

    e) Other, please state

12. The fact that this product provides nursing contact hours influenced my decision to buy it

Strongly disagree   1   2   3   4   5   Strongly agree

13. I found the process of obtaining my continuing education credits for this activity easy to complete

Strongly disagree   1   2   3   4   5   Strongly agree

14. If you did not find the process easy to complete, which of the following areas did you find the most difficult?

    a) Understanding the content of the activity

    b) Understanding the instructions

    c) Completing the exam

    d) Completing the evaluation

    e) Other, please state:

15. How much time did it take for you to complete this activity (including reading the book and completing the exam and the evaluation)? _____

16. If you have any comments on this activity, process, or selection of topics for nursing CE, please note them below.

3

17. Would you be interested in participating as a pilot tester for the development of future HCPro nursing education activities?

    Yes

    No

Thank you for completing this evaluation of our nursing CE activity.